Type 2 Diabetes
in
Children &
ADOLESCENTS

Arlan L. Rosenbloom, MD, and Janet H. Silverstein, MD

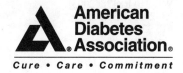

American
Diabetes
Association®

Cure • Care • Commitment

Director, Book Publishing, John Fedor; *Associate Director, Professional Books,* Christine B. Welch; *Editor,* Joyce Raynor; *Associate Director, Book Production,* Peggy M. Rote; *Composition,* Circle Graphics, Inc.; *Cover Design,* SueEllen Lawton; *Printer,* Port City Press, Inc.

Printed in the United States of America
1   3   5   7   9   10   8   6   4   2

The suggestions and information contained in this publication are generally consistent with the *Clinical Practice Recommendations* and other policies of the American Diabetes Association, but they do not represent the policy or position of the Association or any of its boards or committees. Reasonable steps have been taken to ensure the accuracy of the information presented. However, the American Diabetes Association cannot ensure the safety or efficacy of any product or service described in this publication. Individuals are advised to consult a physician or other appropriate health care professional before undertaking any diet or exercise program or taking any medication referred to in this publication. Professionals must use and apply their own professional judgment, experience, and training and should not rely solely on the information contained in this publication before prescribing any diet, exercise, or medication. The American Diabetes Association—its officers, directors, employees, volunteers, and members—assumes no responsibility or liability for personal or other injury, loss, or damage that may result from the suggestions or information in this publication.

⊛ The paper in this publication meets the requirements of the ANSI Standard Z39.48-1992 (permanence of paper).

ADA titles may be purchased for business or promotional use or for special sales. To purchase this book in large quantities, or for custom editions of this book with your logo, contact Lee Romano Sequeira, Special Sales & Promotions, at the address below, or at LRomano@diabetes.org or call 703-299-2046.

American Diabetes Association
1701 North Beauregard Street
Alexandria, Virginia 22311

Library of Congress Cataloging-in-Publication Data

Rosenbloom, Arlan L.
    Type 2 diabetes in children and adolescents : a clinician's guide to diagnosis, epidemiology, pathogenesis, prevention, and treatment / Arlan L. Rosenbloom, Janet H. Silverstein.
        p. ; cm.
    Includes bibliographical references.
    ISBN 1-58040-155-4 (pbk. : alk. paper)
    1. Diabetes in children. 2. Diabetes in adolescence. 3. Non-insulin-dependent diabetes. I. Title: Type II diabetes in children and adolescents. II. Title: Type two diabetes in children and adolescents. III. Silverstein, Janet H., 1944- IV. American Diabetes Association. V. Title.
    [DNLM: 1. Diabetes Mellitus, Non-Insulin-Dependent—Child. 2. Adolescent. WK 810 R8128t 2003]
    RJ420.D5R57 2003
    618.92'462—dc21

                                                            2002033007

Contents

Acknowledgments

We acknowledge the helpful reviews provided by Nathaniel Clark, MD, MS, RD; Kenneth L. Jones, MD; Francine R. Kaufman, MD; and Georgeanna Klingensmith, MD; and the support and inspiration of the diabetes team of the University of Florida Pediatric Endocrine Division.

CHAPTER 1

Introduction

There has been wide recognition in the past decade of the increasing frequency of type 2 diabetes in youth, largely but not exclusively in North America and especially but also not exclusively among Native American, African American, and Hispanic American youth (1–3). An epidemic can be defined simply as an increase in prevalence (i.e., the number of cases in the population) resulting from increased incidence (i.e., the number of cases diagnosed per year). The epidemiologist always asks whether there has been a true increase in incidence or simply an increase in recognition or reporting. Pediatric diabetologists, however, do not doubt that we are witnessing an epidemic of type 2 diabetes in people under 21 years of age (2,4,5).

Although we lack general North American population–based data, such information from the Pima Indian population and from Japan confirm phenomenal increases over the past 20–25 years, and clinic-based data are uniformly alarming (6–8). In some settings, particularly those with a large minority population, newly diagnosed type 2 diabetes is being seen as much or more often than newly diagnosed type 1 diabetes in the 10- to 20-year-old age-group (9).

This is not a newly recognized disease in this population; insulin resistance and occasional type 2 diabetes have been known as complications of childhood obesity for at least 30 years. Harvey Knowles wrote in 1971 (10),

> "A second type of diabetes in young persons closely resembles that of the stable middle-aged onset type. Herein the patients, as a rule, have no symptoms, are overweight, can secrete insulin, and respond to sulfonylurea therapy. Often the diagnosis is made serendipitously. In the Juvenile Diabetic Clinic at the Cincinnati General Hospital, 11 of these patients have been followed along with 300 patients with

the unstable insulin deficient type of diabetes. The age of these 11 patients at diagnosis ranged from 11 to 17 years. The prevalence of this type of diabetes very likely is higher than presently appreciated, because of lack of symptoms or signs leading to suspicion of diabetes."

The concern is not simply that type 2 diabetes threatens to become as frequent as type 1 diabetes in the pediatric population. It is the recognition that type 2 diabetes is a manifestation of the insulin resistance syndrome, which bestows additional cardiovascular risk (11), that youth-onset type 2 diabetes may be associated with greater risk of microvascular disease than even type 1 diabetes (12), that the context and treatment paradigm is more problematic than that for type 1 diabetes, and that the public health implications are consequently more devastating. Compared with patients with type 1 diabetes, young patients with type 2 diabetes are more likely to have single parents with less than a high school education and fewer economic and community resources and, because they are adolescents, are more likely to be influenced by their peers than by their parents or other adults (2,13). For these and other reasons, patients with type 2 diabetes are less likely to be compliant with treatment, and treatment is even more sharply focused on behavior than is treatment for type 1 diabetes. These factors combine to make the risk of early complications even greater in type 2 diabetes than in type 1 diabetes.

This book is part of the continuing response of the American Diabetes Association (ADA) to this serious, emerging public health problem. In late 1998, ADA organized a consensus panel to address the following questions about type 2 diabetes in children and adolescents:

- What is the classification of diabetes in children and adolescents?
- What is the epidemiology?
- What is the pathophysiology?
- Who should be tested?
- How should children and adolescents with type 2 diabetes be treated?
- Can type 2 diabetes in children and adolescents be prevented?

The resulting consensus statement was accepted by a committee of the American Academy of Pediatrics and published simultaneously in *Diabetes Care* (14) and *Pediatrics* (15). Although these questions were addressed by experts with extensive clinical and research experience with type 2 diabetes in children, little of the consensus report was evidence based or data based. There has been substantial funding since then to better understand the pathogenesis, scope, prevention, and treatment of this condition.

Our intention with this book is to put the available information into a readily accessible format for the physician or diabetes educator dealing with this challenging individual and community problem. The book follows the basic structure set forth in the ADA consensus statement. We have chosen to use an outline rather than formal narrative style, which we hope will enhance the accessibility and identification of needed information.

REFERENCES

1. Fagot-Campagna A, Pettitt DJ, Engelgau MM, Burrows MT, Geiss LS, Valdez R, et al.: Type 2 diabetes among North American children and adolescents: an epidemiological review and a public health perspective. *J Pediatr* 136:664–672, 2000
2. Rosenbloom AL: Increasing incidence of type 2 diabetes mellitus in children and adolescents: treatment considerations. *Pediatr Drugs* 4:209–221, 2002
3. Kadiki OA, Reddy MR, Marzouk AA: Incidence of insulin-dependent diabetes (IDDM) and non-insulin-dependent diabetes (NIDDM) (0–34 years at onset) in Benghazi, Libya. *Diabetes Res Clin Pract* 32:165–173, 1996
4. Dabelea-D, Pettitt DJ, Jones KL, Arslanian SA: Type 2 diabetes mellitus in minority children and adolescents. *Endocrinol Metab Clin North Am* 28:709–729, 1999
5. Kaufman FR: Type 2 diabetes mellitus in children and youth: a new epidemic. *J Pediatr Endocrinol Metab* 15 (Suppl. 2):737–744, 2002
6. Dabelea D, Hanson RL, Bennett PH, Roumain J, Knowler WC, Pettitt DJ: Increasing prevalence of type 2 diabetes in American Indian children. *Diabetologia* 41:904–910, 1998
7. Kitagawa T, Owada M, Urakami T, Yamauchi K: Increased incidence of non-insulin dependent diabetes mellitus among Japanese schoolchildren correlates with an increased intake of animal protein and fat. *Clin Pediatr* 37:111–115, 1998
8. Pinhas-Hamiel O, Dolan LM, Daniels SR, Standiford D, Khoury PR, Zeitler P: Increased incidence of non-insulin-dependent diabetes mellitus among adolescents. *J Pediatr* 128:608–615, 1996
9. Neufeld ND, Raffal LF, Landon C, Chen Y-DI, Vadheim CM: Early presentation of type 2 diabetes in Mexican-American youth. *Diabetes Care* 21:80–86, 1998
10. Knowles HC: Diabetes mellitus in childhood and adolescence. *Med Clin North Am* 55:975–987, 1971
11. Hu FB, Stampfer MJ, Haffner SM, Solomon CG, Willett WC, Manson JE: Elevated risk of cardiovascular disease prior to clinical diagnosis of type 2 diabetes. *Diabetes Care* 25:1129–1134, 2002

12. Yokoyama H, Okudaira M, Otani T, Watanabe C, Takaike H, Miuira J, et al.: High incidence of diabetic nephropathy in early-onset Japanese NIDDM patients: risk analysis. *Diabetes Care* 21:1080–1085, 1998
13. Pinhas-Hamiel O, Standiford D, Hamiel D, Dolan LM, Cohen R, Zeitler PS: The type 2 family: a setting for development and treatment of adolescent type 2 diabetes mellitus. *Arch Pediatr Adolesc Med* 153:1063–1067, 1999
14. American Diabetes Association: Type 2 diabetes in children and adolescents (Consensus Statement). *Diabetes Care* 23:381–389, 2000
15. American Diabetes Association: Type 2 diabetes in children and adolescents. *Pediatrics* 105:671–680, 2000

CHAPTER 2

Diagnosis and Classification of Diabetes in Children

DEFINITION

- The diagnosis of diabetes includes a wide array of diseases that are characterized by persistent hyperglycemia (Table 1).
- Insulin is the only physiologically significant hypoglycemic hormone. Therefore, hyperglycemia must be the result of impaired secretion of insulin from the β-cells of the pancreas; resistance to the effect of insulin in the liver, muscle, and fat cells; or a combination of these pathophysiologic situations.
- The current criteria for diabetes include categories of impaired glucose tolerance (IGT) and impaired fasting glucose that are considered to be states of *pre-diabetes*, reflecting an appreciation of the fact that these pre-clinical states are associated with increased cardiovascular morbidity (1).

CLASSIFICATION

Tables 2–6 outline the features of the types of diabetes that need to be considered in children and adolescents, based on what is known of the etiology, in keeping with the American Diabetes Association's Expert Committee on the Diagnosis and Classification of Diabetes Mellitus (1). Contemporary understanding of the pathogenesis of various forms of diabetes made previous classification based on treatment inappropriate.

TABLE 1. Criteria for the Diagnosis of Diabetes

- Symptoms plus random plasma glucose concentration ≥200 mg/dl (11 mmol/l), *or*
- Fasting plasma glucose ≥126 mg/dl (7 mmol/l), *or*
- 2-h plasma glucose ≥200 mg/dl (11 mmol/l) during an oral glucose tolerance test. The test should be performed using a glucose load containing the equivalent of 75 g anhydrous glucose dissolved in water for individuals weighing >43 kg and 1.75 g/kg for individuals weighing ≤43 kg.

In the absence of marked hyperglycemia with decompensation, these criteria should be confirmed by repeat testing on a different day. The oral glucose tolerance test is not recommended for routine clinical use. Impaired glucose tolerance (IGT) is defined by a 2-h plasma glucose level between 140 and 200 mg/dl. Impaired fasting glucose is defined by a level between ≥110 and <126 mg/dl. From the Expert Committee on the Diagnosis and Classification of Diabetes Mellitus (1).

Table 2. Immune Mediated Type 1 Diabetes

- β-Cell destruction, usually leading to absolute insulin deficiency
- Occurs throughout childhood, with as great or greater incidence under 10 years of age as in 10–20 year olds
- Much less frequent in Asians and native North Americans and somewhat less frequent in African-Americans than in those of European origin
- Associated with HLA specificities
- First-degree relatives of 5–10% of patients affected
- Polygenic inheritance
- Equal sex ratio
- Autoantibodies to insulin (IAA), islet cell cytoplasm (ICA), glutamic acid de-hydrogenase (GAD), or tyrosine phosphatase (insulinoma-associated) antibody (IA-2 and IA-2β) at diagnosis in 85–98%
- Ketosis or ketoacidosis common at onset
- Period of weight loss, polyuria, polydipsia, fatigue common; nonspecific symptoms often missed in infants and toddlers
- Signs of insulin resistance, such as hypertension or acanthosis nigricans, absent at diagnosis
- Low to absent insulin secretion, as indicated by C-peptide concentration; however, following initial diagnosis and treatment, partial recovery can last for months to (very rarely) several years

Table 3. Idiopathic Type 1 Diabetes

- May be difficult to distinguish from immune mediated type 1 diabetes
- Includes what is referred to as atypical diabetes mellitus (ADM) or "Flatbush" diabetes, that has been variously considered as a form of type 1 diabetes, type 2 diabetes, or maturity onset diabetes of the young (MODY) (1–5)
  - Occurs throughout childhood, and rarely past age 40
  - Only described in African-American individuals

Table 3. (*Continued*)

- Not associated with HLA specificities
- Strong family history in multiple generations with autosomal dominant pattern of inheritance
- Not associated with obesity beyond that in the general African-American population
- Abnormal sex ratio—M:F 1:3
- No islet autoimmunity
- Ketosis or ketoacidosis common at onset
- Insulin usually not necessary for survival after treatment of acute metabolic deterioration, although diabetic control may be poor and ketoacidosis can recur without insulin treatment in some individuals
- Insulin resistance not characteristic
- Insulin secretion present but diminished, without long-term deterioration of islet cell function

Table 4. Maturity Onset Diabetes of the Young (MODY) (6)

- MODY as a proportion of all diabetes widely variable among different populations, from 0.14% in Germany to 3% in England and 4.8% in Madras, India
- Multigenerational transmission in an autosomal dominant pattern; often necessary to test asymptomatic individuals to demonstrate the presence of diabetes
- Rarely affects racial/ethnic groups other than Caucasians
- Onset subtle, usually before 25 years of age, with insulin usually not being required for treatment
- Molecular defects in 6 genes, involving over 200 different mutations (7)

Table 5. Type 2 Diabetes (8,9)

- Occurs predominantly during second decade of life, mean ~13.5 years, but also in prepubertal children, including as young as 4 years
- Much greater risk in African-American, native North American, Hispanic (especially Mexican)-American, Asian, and South Asian (Indian Peninsula) than in Caucasian individuals
- Not associated with HLA specificities
- 75% or more have first- or second-degree relative affected
- Polygenic inheritance
- Variable sex ratio (M:F) from 1:4–6 in native North Americans to 1:1.7 in African-Americans, 1:1.3 in Mexican-Americans, and 1:1 in Libyan Arabs
- Not usually associated with islet cell autoimmunity
- Ketosis or ketoacidosis in one-third or more of newly diagnosed patients, accounting for most of the misclassification of type 2 diabetes patients as type 1 diabetes patients

(*continued*)

Table 5. (*Continued*)

- Fatal complications of severe dehydration (hyperosmolar hyperglycemic coma, hypokalemia) possible at or before diagnosis
- Often detected in the asymptomatic individual as a result of testing because of risk factors or during routine school or sports examinations
- Insulin resistance, with other features of the insulin resistance syndrome (hyperlipidemia, hypertension, acanthosis nigricans, ovarian hyperandrogenism)
- Highly variable insulin secretion, depending on disease status and duration, from delayed, but markedly elevated, to diminished; 50% reduction in insulin secretory capacity at the time of diagnosis in adults with symptoms, and insulin dependence by 6–7 years later
- Obesity, with body mass index (BMI) above 85th–95th percentile for age and sex

Table 6. Autoantibody Positive Type 2 Diabetes

- ICA and GADA in adults with typical type 2 diabetes, who are referred to as having either type 1.5 or, more commonly, latent autoimmune diabetes of adults (LADA) (10,11)
- United Kingdom Prospective Diabetes Study (10) found that
  - LADA is age related: 21% of individuals 25–34 years old (n = 157) ICA positive, 34% GADA positive, and 20% positive for both antibodies, decreasing to 4%, 7%, and 2%, respectively among those 55–65 years old (n = 1769)
  - antibody positive individuals are significantly less overweight than antibody negative patients
  - glycated hemoglobin A1c (A1C) concentrations are significantly higher in antibody positive individuals
  - β-cell function is significantly less in antibody positive individuals, the most dramatic difference being in the younger patients, resulting in a more rapid development of insulin dependence, usually by 3 years duration
- Swedish study of all individuals 15–34 years old with newly diagnosed diabetes over a two-year period (n = 764) who were tested for ICA, GADA, and IA/2A (11) found
  - 76% classified type 1, 14% type 2, and the rest unclassified
  - 47% of type 2 and 59% of unclassified patients positive for one or more antibodies
  - antibody positive type 2 or unclassifiable patients significantly lighter, with lower C-peptide concentrations, than antibody negative patients
- Comparison of clinical parameters, haplotype and antibody patterns in 57 adults with type 1 diabetes, 54 with LADA, and 190 with type 2 diabetes indicates that LADA is a slowly progressive form of type 1 diabetes, rather than a variant of type 2 diabetes (12), with
  - no difference in BMI, waist:hip ratio, lipid profile, and BP between those with LADA and those with type 1 diabetes

Table 6. (*Continued*)

- lower BMI, waist:hip ratio, lipids, and BP in patients with LADA and type 1 diabetes than in those with type 2 diabetes
- similar baseline C-peptide levels in patients with LADA and type 1 diabetes but a more rapid decline with type 1 diabetes
- similar prevalence of HLA haplotypes associated with high risk for diabetes in LADA and type 1 diabetes
- LADA more commonly associated with presence of a single islet-specific antibody compared to type 1 diabetes
- Study of 48 children with type 2 diabetes (13) found
  - 8% ICA512 (fragment of ICA) positive; 30% GADA positive, 35% IAA positive
  - no correlation of antibody positivity with degree of obesity
  - thyroid autoimmunity in subjects with islet cell autoimmunity
- Study of 37 African-American children and adolescents with type 2 diabetes (14) found
  - 10.8% positive for GADA, IA-2, or both
  - no difference in treatment requirements (oral agent vs. insulin) between positive and negative patients

The accelerator hypothesis has been proposed to explain the development of diabetes-related autoimmunity in typical type 2 diabetes as the result of hyperglycemia secondary to insulin resistance inducing β-cell apoptosis (glucotoxicity) with the development of β-cell autoimmunity (15). Because of the high frequency of evidence of islet cell autoimmunity in otherwise typical type 2 diabetes, particularly in young people, ICA and GADA testing may be worthwhile in all pediatric patients considered to have type 2 diabetes.

- Antibodies will indicate an earlier need for insulin.
- Antibodies will indicate the need to check for thyroid autoimmunity and to consider other associated autoimmune disorders.
- GADA may be the more important predictor of insulin therapy over the short term (3 years) (11).

The characteristic features of the main forms of diabetes seen in children and adolescents are summarized in Table 7.

Uncertainties of Classification

Unfortunately, the distinctions indicated by the features noted above are not as certain as we would like. The clinician is obliged to weigh the evidence

TABLE 7. Classification of the Types of Diabetes Seen in Children

	Type 1 Diabetes	ADM*	MODY	Type 2 Diabetes
Age at onset	Throughout childhood	Pubertal	Pubertal	Pubertal
Predominant ethnicity or ethnic distribution	All (low frequency in Asians)	African-American	Caucasian	Hispanic, African American, Native American
Onset	Acute, severe	Acute, severe	Subtle	Subtle to severe
Islet autoimmunity	Present	Absent	Absent	Absent
Insulin secretion	Very low	Moderately low	Variable	Variable
Insulin sensitivity	Normal (with blood glucose control)	Normal	Normal	Decreased
Ketosis, ketoacidosis at onset	Up to 40%	Common	Rare	Up to 33%
Obesity	As in population	As in population	Uncommon	>90%
Proportion of diabetes	–80%†	>10%	<5%	~20%†
% of probands with affected first- or second-degree relative	5–10%	>75%	100%	~80%
Mode of inheritance	Non-Mendelian, generally sporadic	Autosomal dominant	Autosomal dominant	Non-Mendelian, strongly familial

*ADM, atypical diabetes mellitus, also known as "Flatbush" diabetes, which may be classified as idiopathic type 1 diabetes (1).
†The proportion of pediatric diabetes patients with ADM, MODY, or type 2 diabetes will vary with the ethnic mix of the population; the proportion of type 2 diabetes is increasing.
Adapted from Winter et al. (6) and Rosenbloom et al. (8).

in an individual patient for distinguishing between type 1 and type 2 diabetes. There are several reasons for this conundrum.

- With increasing obesity in childhood, as many as 20–25% of newly diagnosed type 1 diabetes patients may be obese (16). This will also be true with ADM.

■ Type 2 diabetes is common in the general population, with a random family history likelihood of ~15% or greater in minority populations, reducing the specificity of this characteristic.

■ Positive family history for type 2 diabetes is increased for patients with type 1 diabetes as much as threefold over that of the nondiabetic population, and type 1 diabetes is more frequent in relatives of patients with type 2 diabetes (17).

■ Genetic interaction between type 1 diabetes and type 2 diabetes is further suggested by HLA haplotype interaction (18) and the finding of islet autoimmunity markers at onset in some children and adults with typical type 2 diabetes, as noted above.

■ There is considerable overlap in insulin or C-peptide measurements at onset of diabetes and over the first year or so in type 1 and type 2 diabetes because of the recovery phase of autoimmune diabetes (the honeymoon) and the degree of glucotoxicity/lipotoxicity impairing insulin secretion at the time of testing. Elevated C-peptide levels are indicative of type 2 diabetes, but normal concentrations, or suppressed levels in the presence of hyperglycemia, are not diagnostic.

■ One-third or more of pediatric patients with type 2 diabetes have ketonuria or ketoacidosis at diagnosis (9,19,20).

What Is the Magnitude of Possible Misclassification?

■ Among ~700 patients 5–19 years old at three university centers in Florida newly diagnosed over a 5-year period from 1994 to 1999, 3% of those initially classified as having type 1 diabetes (17 of 605) were later diagnosed with type 2 diabetes, and 8% of those initially diagnosed with type 2 diabetes were reclassified as having type 1 diabetes (6 of 77) (21).

■ With increasing awareness of type 2 diabetes in children, the Florida experience probably reflects the true magnitude of the diagnostic problem.

DIAGNOSTIC STRATEGY

Features helpful in differentiating type 1 and type 2 diabetes in children and adolescents are summarized in Table 8.

Acute Onset

■ Nonobese individuals who are not African American are very likely to have type 1 diabetes and seldom require further testing.

TABLE 8. Differentiating Type 1 from Type 2 Diabetes in Children and Adolescents

	Type 1 Diabetes	Type 2 Diabetes	Comment
Demographic characteristics			
Family history	3–5%	74–100%	Extensive family history suggests type 2 diabetes; type 2 diabetes affects minorities disproportionately
Age or pubertal status	Variable	>10 or pubertal*	Type 1 diabetes can occur at any age; only 10% of children with type 2 diabetes are younger than 10 years of age or prepubertal
Sex	F = M	F > M	Some sex differences in type 2 diabetes may reflect differences in the use of medical care
Presentation			
Asymptomatic	Rare	Common	Type 2 diabetes often detected incidentally on routine physical examination
Symptom duration	Days or weeks	Weeks or months	Predominant symptoms are polyuria, polydipsia, polyphagia, and nocturia
Weight loss	Common	Common	Children with type 2 diabetes may lose as many or more pounds; children with type 1 diabetes usually lose a greater percentage of body weight
Hyperglycemic hyperosmolar state	Very rare	Occurs	Children with type 2 diabetes can develop severe, fatal dehydration and electrolyte disturbance (22)
Physical findings			
BMI at diagnosis	≤75th percentile	≥85th percentile	Individuals with BMIs in the 75–85th percentile often present greatest diagnostic challenge
Acanthosis nigricans	No	Common	Useful marker in hyperglycemic child
Biochemistry at diagnosis			
Hyperglycemia	Variable	Variable	Degree of hyperglycemia at diagnosis is not useful in delineating diabetes type
Ketosis and ketonuria	Common	Moderately common	Not useful for diagnosis of diabetes type

TABLE 8. *(Continued)*

	Type 1 Diabetes	Type 2 Diabetes	Comment
Acidosis	Common	Moderately common	Not useful for diagnosis of diabetes type
Other markers			
A1C	Elevated	Elevated	Not useful for diagnosis of diabetes type
Insulin or C-peptide/serum	Low (may be nl early)	Normal-high	Hyperinsulinism reflects insulin resistance; low levels may be found in children with type 2 diabetes at diagnosis; repeat testing 3–6 months after diagnosis may find elevated levels
Autoimmune markers	Common	Uncommon	Includes anti–islet cell antibodies and anti-GADAs; absence does not rule out type 1 diabetes

*Occasionally in the 8- to 10-year-old age-group and as young as 4 years of age. Adapted from Hale DE: Type 2 diabetes: an increasing pediatric problem. Unpublished.

- Nonobese African American youths with a three-generation history of diabetes suggestive of autosomal-dominant transmission and without islet cell autoimmunity markers likely have ADM.
- In obese patients, islet cell autoimmunity testing should be considered. If this is not practical, or if the patient has acanthosis nigricans, the diagnosis can usually be clarified during the first several months by reducing and, if glycemic goals obtained, stopping acutely required insulin, with weight reduction, exercise, and, as necessary, oral hypoglycemic therapy.

Insidious Onset

- Obese individuals who are not African American or who are African American but do not have a three-generation history of early-onset diabetes in a dominant pattern can be considered to have type 2 diabetes.
- Islet autoantibody testing will be helpful in a lean patient. The presence of antibodies indicates type 1 diabetes picked up early; the absence of antibodies may indicate MODY.

- Because MODY is rare, routine testing for the various mutations that have been described is not of value.
- Fasting C-peptide or insulin measurements, if insulin treatment has not been given, may be of value after stabilization; elevated levels are indicative of type 2 diabetes. Repeat testing at 1 year or later may be needed for individuals with normal results.

REFERENCES

1. Expert Committee on the Diagnosis and Classification of Diabetes Mellitus: Report of the Expert Committee on the Diagnosis and Classification of Diabetes Mellitus. *Diabetes Care* 24:S5–S20, 2001
2. Winter WE, Maclaren NK, Riley WJ, Clarke DW, Kappy MS, Spillar RP: Maturity onset diabetes of youth in black Americans. *N Engl J Med* 316:285–291, 1987
3. Banerji MA, Leibovitz H: Insulin sensitive and insulin resistant variants in IDDM. *Diabetes* 38:784–792, 1989
4. Banerji MA, Chaiken RL, Huey H, Tuomi T, Norin AJ, Mackay IR, et al.: GAD antibody negative NIDDM in adult black subjects with diabetic keto-acidosis and increased frequency of human leukocyte antigen DR3 and DR4: Flatbush diabetes. *Diabetes* 43:741–745, 1994
5. Banerji MA: Impaired beta-cell and alpha-cell function in African-American children with type 2 diabetes mellitus: "Flatbush diabetes." *J Pediatr Endocrinol Metab* 15 (Suppl. 1):493-501, 2002
6. Winter WE, Nakamura M, House DV: Monogenic diabetes mellitus in youth: the MODY syndromes. *Endocrinol Metab Clin North Am* 28:765–785, 1999
7. Doria A, Plengvidhya N: Recent advances in the genetics of maturity onset diabetes of the young and other forms of autosomal dominant diabetes. *Curr Opin Endocrinol Diabetes* 7:203–210, 2000
8. Rosenbloom AL, Joe JR, Young RS, Winter WE: The emerging epidemic of type 2 diabetes mellitus in youth. *Diabetes Care* 22:345–354, 1999
9. American Diabetes Association: Type 2 diabetes in children and adolescents (Consensus Statement). *Diabetes Care* 23:381–389, 2000
10. Turner R, Stratton I, Horton V, Manley S, Zimmet P, Mackay IR, Shattock M, Bottazzo GF, Holman R, for the UK Prospective Diabetes Study (UKPDS) Group: UKPDS 25: autoantibodies to islet cell cytoplasm and glutamic acid decarboxylase for prediction of insulin requirement in type 2 diabetes. *Lancet* 350:1288–1293, 1997
11. Landin-Olsson M: Latent autoimmune diabetes in adults. *Ann N Y Acad Sci* 958:112–116, 2002

12. Hosszúfalusi N, Vatay Á, Rajczy K, Prohászka Z, Pozsonyi É, Horváth L, Grosz A, Gerő L, Madácsy L, Romics L, Karádi I, Füst G, Pánczél P: Similar genetic features and different islet cell autoantibody pattern of latent autoimmune diabetes in adults (lada) compared with adult-onset type 1 diabetes with rapid progression. *Diabetes Care* 26:452–457, 2003

13. Hathout EH, Thomas W, El-Shahawy M, Nabab F, Mace JW: Diabetic autoimmune markers in children and adolescents with type 2 diabetes. *Pediatrics* 107:E102, 2001

14. Umpaichitra V, Banerji MA, Castells S: Autoantibodies in children with type 2 diabetes mellitus. *J Pediatr Endocrinol Metab* 15:525–530, 2002

15. Wilkin TJ: The accelerator hypothesis. *Diabetologia* 44:914–922, 2001

16. Strauss RS, Pollack HA: Epidemic increase in childhood overweight, 1986–1998. *JAMA* 286:2845–2848, 2001

17. Dahlquist G, Blom L, Tuvemo T, Nystrom L, Sandstrom A, Wall S: The Swedish childhood diabetes study: results from a nine-year case register and a one-year case-referent study indicating that type 1 (insulin-dependent) diabetes mellitus is associated with both type 2 (non-insulin-dependent) diabetes mellitus and autoimmune disorders. *Diabetologia* 32:2–6, 1989

18. Li H, Lindholm E, Almgren P, Gustafsson A, Forsblom C, Groop L, Tuomi T: Possible human leukocyte antigen-mediated genetic interaction between type 1 and type 2 diabetes. *J Clin Endocrinol Metab* 86:574–582, 2001

19. Pinhas-Hamiel O, Dolan LM, Zeitler PS: Diabetic ketoacidosis among obese African American adolescents with NIDDM. *Diabetes Care* 28:484–486, 1997

20. Sellers EAC, Dean H: Diabetic ketoacidosis: a complication of type 2 diabetes in Canadian aboriginal youth. *Diabetes Care* 23:1202–1204, 2000

21. Macaluso CJ, Bauer UE, Deeb LC, Malone JI, Chaudhari M, Silverstein J, Eidson M, Arbelaez AM, Goldberg RB, Gaughan-Bailey B, Brooks RG, Rosenbloom AL: Type 2 diabetes mellitus among Florida children and adolescents, 1994 through 1998. *Public Health Reports* 117:373–379, 2002

22. Morales A, Rosenbloom AL: Death at the onset of type 2 diabetes (T2DM) in African-American youth. *Pediatr Res* 51:124A, 2002

CHAPTER 3

Epidemiology of Type 2 Diabetes and Obesity in Children

EVIDENCE FOR AN EPIDEMIC OF TYPE 2 DIABETES IN CHILDREN (TABLES 9–11)

North America

- In the Pima Indian population, in which 50% of adults have type 2 diabetes
  - in 1979, prevalence of type 2 diabetes was
    - 1% (9 of 1,000) of those age 15–24 years
    - nil in those younger than 15 years (1)
  - by the 1990s, type 2 diabetes prevalence was
    - 5% of those 15–19 years old (51 of 1,000)
    - 2.2% of those 10–14 years old (22 of 1,000) (2)
- First Nation population in Canada: The frequency of type 2 diabetes in children and youth was comparable to that of type 1 diabetes in Caucasians (3)
- Review of 1,027 consecutive records of children 0–19 years old diagnosed with diabetes in Cincinnati, Ohio found (4)
  - 2–4% diagnosed with type 2 diabetes from 1982 to 1992 (stable for over 20 years; Knowles [5] reported that ~3.5% of patients in this same clinic had type 2 diabetes in 1971)
  - 16% diagnosed with type 2 diabetes in 1994
  - 33% of newly diagnosed patients age 10–19 years with type 2 diabetes in 1994

Table 9. Estimates of the Frequency of Type 2 Diabetes in Children and Adolescents

Location	Race/ethnicity	Year	Age (years)	Incidence per 10^5	Prevalence per 10^3	% of All DM	M:F
Arizona	Pima Indian	1979	<15	0	0	—	—
			15–24	—	9	—	—
		1996	10–14	—	22.3	—	—
			15–19	—	50.9	—	1:5
Manitoba	First Nation		5–14	—	1	—	1:4
Ontario	First Nation		<16	—	2.3	—	1:6
Cincinnati	Caucasian, African American	1971	0–19	—	—	3.5	—
		1994	0–19	—	—	16	—
			10–19	7.2	—	33	1:1.7
California	Mexican-American	1994	0–17	—	—	45	1:1.3
Libya	Arab	1990	10–14	1.8	—	22	1:1
			15–19	5.9	—	39	1:2
Tokyo	Japanese	1980	6–11	0.2	—	—	—
			12–15	7.2	—	—	—
		1995	6–11	2.0	—	—	1:2
			12–15	13.9	—	—	1:1.2
Taiwan	Chinese	1993–1995	6–18	10	—	—	1:1.5
Bangladesh	Asian Indian	1997	15–19	—	0.6	—	—

- estimated age-specific incidence to be 7.2 per 100,000,
  - one-half the incidence rate for type 1 diabetes in the childhood population
  - a tenfold increase since 1982
- Cincinnati (4) and Arkansas (6): African Americans accounted for 70–75% of pediatric type 2 diabetes patients.
- Mexican Americans (7): One-third of diabetes patients under the age of 17 years have type 2 diabetes.
- In a study of 682 patients age 5–19 years diagnosed between January 1, 1994, and December 31, 1998, at the three university diabetes centers in Florida (8)

- 86% were considered to have type 1 diabetes and 14% type 2 diabetes
- 47% of patients with type 1 diabetes and 63% of patients with type 2 diabetes were female
- only 46% of those with type 2 diabetes were African American, 22% were Hispanic, and the rest were non-Hispanic Caucasian
- the proportion of newly diagnosed patients with diabetes who had type 2 diabetes increased from 8.7% in 1994 to 19% in 1998

Table 10. Type 2 Diabetes in Children and Adolescents Outside of North America

- Libyan Arabs (9)
  - Age-specific annual incidence
    - 6/100,000 for age 15–19 years
    - 26/100,000 for age 20–24 years
    - 100/100,000 for age 25–29 years
    - 240/100,000 for age 30–34 years
  - Overall (age 0–34)
    - >2 times the incidence of type 1 diabetes in males
    - >4 times the incidence of type 1 diabetes in females
- Hong Kong Chinese (10)
  - Accounts for >90% of young onset diabetes in Chinese
  - Strongly familial
  - Associated with obesity
- Taiwan Chinese (11)
  - From 1992 to 1999, annual urine screening of schoolchildren followed by repeat test and fasting blood test for glycemia, as indicated
  - Nearly 3 million students tested each semester
  - Incidence rates
    - 8.3 per 100,000 among boys and 12.0 per 100,000 among girls
    - significant increase from 6th grade for boys and 4th grade for girls, with peak rates
      - 14.7 per 100,000 in 8th grade for boys
      - 19.0 per 100,000 in 6th grade for girls
- Japanese (12)
  - Type 1 diabetes relatively rare as in Chinese
  - Annual urine testing of schoolchildren within Tokyo prefecture since 1975, followed by oral glucose tolerance testing as indicated
    - ~4 fold increased incidence of type 2 diabetes between 1976 and 1995
    - increased incidence of type 2 diabetes paralleled by increasing obesity rates

(continued)

Table 10. (*Continued*)

- Bangladeshi (13)
  - Population sampling of ~7000 suburban residents including ~300 age 15–20 years
  - Type 2 diabetes prevalence 0.6/1000
  - Type 2 diabetes associated with increased BMI
- Australian Aborigines (14)
  - 74 children and adolescents followed for 5 years
  - Increase in prevalence of overweight from 2.7% to 17.6% over the 5 years
  - At end of study (mean age 18.5 years) 8% with impaired glucose tolerance, 2.7% with type 2 diabetes and 22% with elevated cholesterol
- New Zealand Maoris (15)
  - 5% of 1,052 diabetes patients diagnosed before age 30, of which 55% were type 2
  - Micro-albuminuria more common in type 2 diabetes (62%) vs. type 1 diabetes (18%)
  - 86% of patients with type 2 diabetes overweight vs. 44% of those with type 1 diabetes
  - Female:male 1.5:1

THE EPIDEMIC OF OBESITY

United States

- Obesity, defined in adults as a BMI ≥30 kg/m^2, doubled in frequency in the adult population in the last decade of the 20th century (16).
- Obesity prevalence in 2000 was ~20% of adults (16):
  - 18.5% of Caucasians
  - 29.3% of African Americans
  - 23.4% of Hispanics
- The National Health and Nutrition Examination Survey (NHANES) III conducted between 1988 and 1994 described a doubling in prevalence of childhood obesity since the 1980s (17).
- NHANES III update of 1999 (18) found BMI >95% for age and sex, varying with ethnicity, in
  - 11–18% of boys 6–11 years old
  - 10–17% of girls 6–11 years old
  - 11–14% of boys 12–19 years old
  - 10–17% of girls 12–19 years old
- The Bogalusa Heart Study, a 20-year (1973–1994), biracial, community-based study in Louisiana of 11,564 individuals 5–24 years old (19):
  - Mean weight increased 0.2 kg/year, and skinfold thickness increased.

- The frequency of overweight doubled.
  - □ Overweight (>85th percentile BMI) increased from 15 to 30%.
  - □ Obesity (>95th percentile BMI) increased from 5 to 11% in those 5–14 years old and from 5 to 15% in those age 15–17 years old.
- Increases in the second 10 years of the study were 50% greater than those in the first 10 years.

■ The National Longitudinal Survey of Youth, a prospective cohort study of 8,270 children age 4–12 years (22):
  - There was a significant increase in "overweight" (>95th percentile of BMI for age and sex) and risk of overweight (85th–95th percentile of BMI).
  - Prevalence rates in 1998 (Fig. 1) were
    - □ BMI >85th percentile: African Americans 38.4%, Hispanics 37.9%, Caucasians 25.8%
    - □ BMI >95th percentile: African Americans 21.5%, Hispanics 21.8%, Caucasians 12.3%

International

Table 11. Obesity Trends in Children and Youth Outside of the United States

■ Russia—1992 (20)
  - ~7000 patients age 6–18 years examined
  - 6% obese (>95th percentile BMI), 10% overweight (85th–95th percentile) using U.S. BMI reference data
■ China—1993 (20)
  - ~3000 patients age 6–18 years examined
  - 3.6% obese, 3.4% overweight (as defined above)
■ United Kingdom—1996 (21)
  - 22% overweight, 10% obese at age 6 years
  - 31% overweight, 17% obese at age 15 years
■ Europe (21): highest rates of childhood obesity in Eastern Europe (particularly Hungary), and Spain, Italy, and Greece

REFERENCES

1. Savage PJ, Bennett PH, Senter RG, Miller M: High prevalence of diabetes in young Pima Indians. *Diabetes* 28:937–942, 1979
2. Dabelea D, Hanson RL, Bennett PH, Roumain J, Knowler WC, Pettitt DJ: Increasing prevalence of type 2 diabetes in American Indian children. *Diabetologia* 41:904–910, 1998

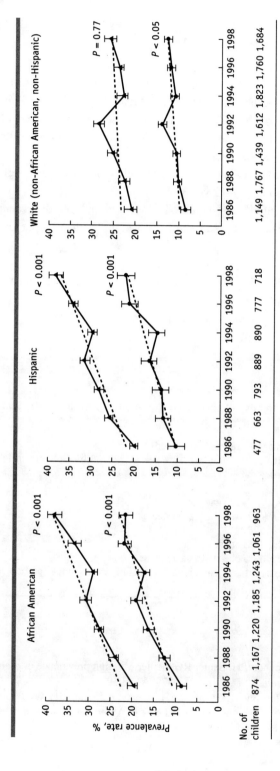

FIGURE 1. Prevalence rates of BMIs >95th percentile. Weighted sample. In each graph, the dashed line and significance value represent linearized trends for each subgroup after adjustment for the child's age. ▲, BMI >85th percentile; ●, BMI >95th percentile. From U.S. Department of Labor, Bureau of Labor Statistics (22).

3. Dean HJ: NIDDM-Y in First Nation children in Canada. *Clin Pediatr* 39:89–96, 1998

4. Pinhas-Hamiel O, Dolan LM, Daniels SR, Standiford D, Khoury PR, Zeitler P: Increased incidence of non-insulin-dependent diabetes mellitus among adolescents. *J Pediatr* 128:608–615, 1996

5. Knowles HC: Diabetes mellitus in childhood and adolescence. *Med Clin North Am* 55:975–987, 1971

6. Scott CR, Smith JM, Cradock MM, Pihoker C: Characteristics of youth-onset non-insulin-dependent diabetes mellitus at diagnosis. *Pediatrics* 100:84–91, 1997

7. Neufeld ND, Raffal LF, Landon C, Chen Y-DI, Vadheim CM: Early presentation of type 2 diabetes in Mexican-American youth. *Diabetes Care* 21:80–86, 1998

8. Macaluso CJ, Bauer UE, Deeb LC, Malone JI, Chaudhari M, Silverstein J, Eidson M, Arbelaez AM, Goldberg RB, Gaughan-Bailey B, Brooks RG, Rosenbloom AL: Type 2 diabetes mellitus among Florida children and adolescents, 1994 through 1998. *Public Health Reports* 117:373–379, 2002

9. Kadiki OA, Reddy MR, Marzouk AA: Incidence of insulin-dependent diabetes (IDDM) and non-insulin-dependent diabetes (NIDDM) (0–34 years at onset) in Benghazi, Libya. *Diabetes Res Clin Pract* 32:165–173, 1996

10. Chan JC, Cheung CK, Swaminathan R, Nicholls MG, Cockram CS: Obesity, albuminuria, and hypertension among Hong Kong Chinese with non-insulin-dependent diabetes mellitus (NIDDM). *Postgrad Med J* 69:204–210, 1993

11. Wei JN, Sung FC, Li CY, Chang CH, Lin RS, Lin CC, Chiang CC, Chuang LM: Low birth weight and high birth weight infants are both at an increased risk to have type 2 diabetes among schoolchildren in Taiwan. *Diabetes Care* 26:343–348, 2003

12. Kitagawa T, Owada M, Urakami T, Yamauchi K: Increased incidence of non-insulin dependent diabetes mellitus among Japanese schoolchildren correlates with an increased intake of animal protein and fat. *Clin Pediatr* 37:111–115, 1998

13. Sayeed MA, Hussain MZ, Banu A, Rumi MAK, Azad Khan AK: Prevalence of diabetes in a suburban population of Bangladesh. *Diabetes Res Clin Pract* 34:149–155, 1997

14. Braun B, Zimmerman MB, Kretchmer N, Spargo RM, Smith RM, Gracey M: Risk factors for diabetes and cardiovascular disease in young Australian aborigines: a 5-year follow-up study. *Diabetes Care* 19:472–479, 1996

15. McGrath NM, Parker GN, Dawson P: Early presentation of type 2 diabetes mellitus in young New Zealand Maori. *Diabetes Res Clin Pract* 43:205–209, 1999

16. Mokdad AH, Bowman BA, Ford ES, Vinicor F, Marks JS, Koplan JP: The continuing epidemics of obesity and diabetes in the United States. *JAMA* 286:1195–1200, 2001

17. Strauss RS, Pollack HA: Epidemic increase in childhood overweight, 1986–1998. *JAMA* 286:2845–2848, 2001

18. Centers for Disease Control and Prevention, National Center for Health Statistics: Overweight Among U.S. Children and Adolescents. *National Health and Nutrition Examination Survey* http://www.CDC.gov/NCHS/NHANES.htm

19. Freedman DS, Srinivasan SR, Valdez RA, Williamson DF, Berenson GS: Secular increases in relative weight and obesity among children over two decades: the Bogalusa Heart Study. *Pediatrics* 99:420–426, 1997

20. Wang Y: Cross-national comparison of childhood obesity: the epidemic and the relationship between obesity and socioeconomic status. *Int J Epidemiol* 30:1129–1136, 2001

21. Livingstone B: Epidemiology of childhood obesity in Europe. *Eur J Pediatr* 159 (Suppl. 1):S14–S34, 2000

22. U.S. Department of Labor, Bureau of Labor Statistics. *National Longitudinal Survey of Youth, 1986–1997.* Washington, DC: GPO, 1997

CHAPTER 4

Causes of the Insulin Resistance Syndrome and Type 2 Diabetes

METABOLIC PATHOLOGY

- Insulin resistance is defined as the impairment of the response to the physiological effects of insulin, including those on glucose, lipid, and protein metabolism and on vascular endothelial function.
- Normal glycemic control requires
  - sensing of the glucose concentration by β-cells
  - synthesis and release of insulin
  - binding of insulin to receptors
  - postreceptor function activation:
    - □ increased glucose uptake by muscles, fat, and liver
    - □ decreased glucose production by the liver
- Metabolic defects in type 2 diabetes include
  - peripheral insulin resistance in muscle and fat tissue
  - decreased pancreatic insulin secretion (estimated at 50% of normal by the time of clinical onset in adults)
  - increased hepatic glucose output

Figures 2 and 3 depict the development and natural history of type 2 diabetes.

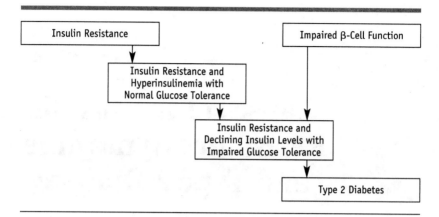

FIGURE 2. Development of type 2 diabetes. Both insulin resistance and impaired β-cell function are required for the development of type 2 diabetes. Adapted from Saltiel AR, Olefsky JM: Thiazolidinediones in the treatment of insulin resistance and type II diabetes. *Diabetes* 45:1661–1669, 1996.

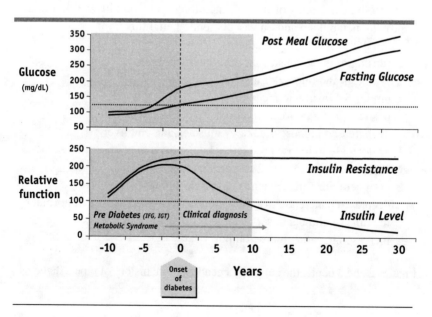

FIGURE 3. Natural history of type 2 diabetes. Kendall DM, Bergenstal RM © 2003 International Diabetes Center, Minneapolis, MN. Used with permission. All rights reserved.

- During the preclinical phase of type 2 diabetes, glycemia is normal, but the insulin response is elevated in response to a standard glucose load or meal or to a glucose clamp.
- As acute insulin response fails to compensate for the insulin resistance, postprandial hyperglycemia develops, followed by fasting hyperglycemia.
- By 6–8 years of overt diabetes, there is usually inadequate β-cell function to permit treatment without supplemental insulin in these adult patients (1). The time course of β-cell decline in children is unknown.

GENETIC BASIS FOR INSULIN RESISTANCE AND TYPE 2 DIABETES

- The epidemic of obesity, together with the ease of gaining weight but the difficulty of losing it, suggests that there may have been a selective advantage to this metabolic phenotype during human evolution.
  - An enhanced ability to store energy as fat would provide survival advantage during the feast or famine existence of hunter-gatherers who expended enormous energy in the quest for food and safety.
  - This phenotype would then become detrimental in the absence of famine and with the enormous reduction in energy expenditure required for daily living.
- Type 2 diabetes would not have developed in predisposed individuals in the absence of opportunities to become obese.
- The *thrifty genotype* hypothesis explains the insulin resistance and relative β-cell insufficiency associated with the development of type 2 diabetes as an adaptation to conserve energy in times of famine (2,3).
- Changes in gene frequency or in the genetic pool cannot explain the rapid increases in type 2 diabetes prevalence within one or two generations in some populations, emphasizing the importance of environmental factors operating against this genetic background.

Evidence that Type 2 Diabetes Is a Genetic Disease (4)

- Family clustering/segregation analysis shows that siblings of affected individuals have 3.5 times the risk of the general population.
- In monozygotic twins, concordance is 80–100%, more than twice the concordance in dizygotic twins.
- Insulin sensitivity and frequency of type 2 diabetes varies by ethnicity.

Types of Inheritance

■ Almost all diabetes in children and adults is polygenic.
■ Monogenic forms provide insight for the study of typical type 2 diabetes (5,6).
  ● Autosomal-dominant forms include MODY and ADM; >200 molecular defects affecting six different genes have been identified in families with MODY.
  ● Maternally inherited (mitochondrial) monogenic forms are characterized by
    □ disease transmission that occurs exclusively from the mother because mitochondria are inherited via the cytoplasm of the ovum
    □ diabetes that is usually indistinguishable from typical type 2 diabetes
    □ affected individuals that also have, in addition to type 2 diabetes, sensorineural hearing loss, cardiomyopathy, optic neuropathy, myopathy, encephalopathy, lactic acidosis, stroke-like syndrome, or epilepsy

Identifying Type 2 Diabetes Susceptibility Genes (5,6)

■ Candidate gene approach
  ● Identifying/choosing an appropriate candidate is problematic.
  ● The candidate may be unknown at the time of the study (e.g., MODY genes, *NIDDM1*, calpain-10).
■ Genome scan approach
  ● The entire genome is scanned for linkages (in families) or associations (in populations).
  ● Microsatellites are particularly useful.
  ● Microassays of mRNA are useful in identifying gene patterns that are overexpressed or underexpressed in specific disease states.
■ Some candidate genes are illustrated in the β-cell–target cell interaction diagram in Figure 4 (7).
■ Over 20 loci have been linked to or associated with type 2 diabetes in adults, varying from population to population.
■ The most important locus identified thus far is *NIDDM1* among Mexican American sibships from Starr County, Texas (8):
  ● population 97% Mexican American
  ● highest disease-specific diabetes mortality rate in Texas
  ● gene pool 31% Native American
  ● 170 affected sibships studied, including 300 siblings with diabetes and 78 without

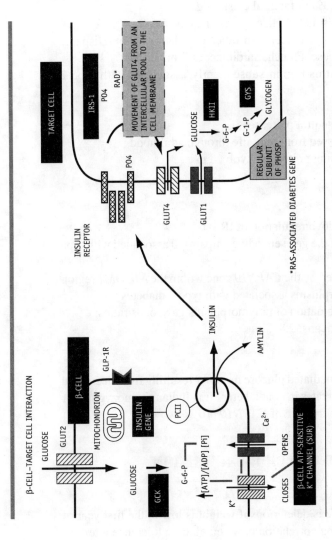

FIGURE 4. Potential sites of genetic defects resulting in type 2 diabetes. β-Cell candidate genes in diabetes include GLUT2 (glucose transporter 2), which is responsible for the facilitative uptake of glucose by β-cells; glucokinase (GCK), which is the β-cell glucose sensor; mitochondrial genes, which provide power to the β-cell (an increased ratio of ATP to ADP + Pi [{ATP}]/[{ADP} + {Pi}]); the ATP-sensitive potassium (K⁺) channel (the sulfonylurea receptor [SUR]); GLP-1R (the β-cell glucagon-like peptide-1 receptor), which responds to GLP from the gastrointestinal tract; insulin; PCII (prohormone convertase II, an example of an insulin-processing protein); and amylin, which is cosecreted with insulin. At the target cell (muscle, fat, or liver), candidate genes include the insulin receptor; intracellular proteins that are phosphorylated (insulin receptor substrate-1 [IRS-1]); GLUT1; hexokinase II, which catalyzes the conversion of glucose to glucose-6-phosphate (G-6-P); glycogen synthase (GYS), which regulates glycogen production; and the regulatory subunit of phosphorylase (PHOSP), which regulates glycogen breakdown. GLUT4 is also a candidate gene, but GLUT4 is expressed only in muscle and fat tissue and is not expressed in the liver. From Rosenbloom et al. (7). Reprinted with permission.

29

- examined 474 autosomal markers and 16 X-linked markers
- *NIDDM1*
  - site on chromosome 2 linked to type 2 diabetes
  - logarithm of odds (LOD) score 3.20
  - accounted for ~30% of familial clustering
  - importance equals that of HLA in type 1 diabetes
  - not linked to type 2 diabetes in other populations (non-Hispanic Caucasian, Japanese, French, Sardinian, or Finnish) (4)
  - calpain gene in this region subsequently associated with type 2 diabetes (9)
- Calpains:
  - calcium-activated neutral proteases
  - ubiquitously expressed from fetal life through adulthood
  - function as processing proteases involved in
    - signaling
    - proliferation
    - differentiation
    - insulin-induced downregulation of IRS-1
  - genetic variation of the gene encoding calpain-10 associated with type 2 diabetes (9)
    - calpain-10 encoded by the *CAPN10* gene within the *NIDDM1* region
    - multiple polymorphisms associated with type 2 diabetes
    - highest risk combination of polymorphisms gave odds ratios:
      - Mexican Americans: 2.8–3.6
      - Finns: 2.6
      - Germans: 5.0
    - reduced insulin-mediated glucose turnover resulting from decreased glucose oxidation rates in nondiabetic Pima Indians homozygous for a common polymorphism of *CAPN10* (10)

ROLE OF FETAL AND CHILDHOOD NUTRITION

Studies in Adults

- High BMI in adult life is deleterious if weight is low in the first year of life. There was a strong correlation between glucose tolerance after age 64 years and weight at 1 year of age in England (11).
- Low birth weight is also associated with an increased risk of type 2 diabetes, with a sevenfold greater risk in individuals with the lowest birth weights compared to those with highest birth weights (also in England [12]).

■ Low birth weight for length was associated with a threefold increased risk of diabetes at age 60 years in Swedish men (13).

■ Low birth weight was associated with a twofold risk of diabetes in 23,000 healthy men from the United States (14).

■ Greater than normal and less than normal birth weight was associated with an increase in adult diabetes risk among Pima Indians (15).

■ Thirty-three-year-old subjects whose mothers smoked during pregnancy were at increased risk for both obesity and diabetes according to a large British longitudinal study (16). This may be the result of the association between smoking and low birth weight or be a direct toxic effect.

■ Twenty-five-year-old subjects born with intrauterine growth retardation (IUGR) ($n = 26$) were compared to 25 control subjects for insulin sensitivity (peripheral glucose uptake) and free fatty acid (FFA) concentrations with a euglycemic-hyperinsulinemic clamp (17):
  ● Despite comparable BMI between groups, those with IUGR had a significantly greater percent body fat.
  ● Insulin-stimulated glucose uptake was significantly lower in IUGR, even after adjustment for BMI, total body fat, or waist-to-hip ratio (as a measure of visceral adiposity).
  ● FFA suppression by insulin was also decreased.
  ● These abnormalities were not associated with changes in first-phase insulin release in response to intravenous glucose, suggesting an early stage of insulin resistance.

Studies in Children and Youth

■ 3,061 Pima Indians age 5–29 years (15):
  ● Current weight correlated with birth weight.
  ● Two-hour glucose testing in those >10 years of age had a U-shaped relationship with birth weight, i.e., higher blood glucose levels in individuals with greater than normal and less than normal birth weight, unrelated to current weight.

■ 477 8-year-old Indian children (18):
  ● Increased cardiovascular risk factors, i.e., hypertension, hyperlipidemia, were associated with low birth weight.
  ● Highest risk was with low birth weight and high-fat mass at 8 years.
  ● Results were thought to reflect fetal undernutrition (see thrifty phenotype below).

■ 139 Caucasian and African American children age 4–14 years who had low birth weight (19):

- Measurements included fasting glucose, insulin, lipids and insulin action and secretion by a tolbutamide-modified frequently sampled intravenous glucose tolerance test; and body composition by dual-energy X-ray absorptiometry and computed tomography.
- Measures were repeated for >1 year (average four times per year).
- Low birth weight was significantly associated with increased fasting insulin and visceral fat mass, less acute insulin response and β-cell function, and lower HDL cholesterol in African American children.
- There were significant differences in measures of insulin sensitivity and HDL between Caucasians and African Americans (thrifty genotype?).
- 429 subjects with type 2 diabetes detected in the Taiwan school screening program (1992–1997) and 549 controls with normal fasting glucose (20):
  - Analyses were adjusted for age, sex, BMI, family history of diabetes, and socioeconomic status.
  - Odds ratios for type 2 diabetes were 2.91 for children with low birth weight (<2,500 grams) and 1.78 for those with high birth weight (≥4,000 grams).
  - Those with type 2 diabetes who had high birth weight were more likely to have a higher BMI and diastolic blood pressure and a family history of diabetes compared with those with low birth weight.

Explanations for the Influence of Birth Weight on Insulin Sensitivity

- Thrifty phenotype hypothesis: Poor nutrition in fetal and early infant life is detrimental to the development and function of the β-cells and insulin-sensitive tissues (primarily muscle), which leads to insulin resistance.
- Thrifty genotype hypothesis: Genetically programmed defective insulin action in utero results in decreased fetal growth and obesity-induced IGT in later childhood or adulthood.

Genetic Factors Affecting Birth Weight that Suggest a Relationship to Glucose Metabolism

- Polymorphism of the VNTR (variable number of tandem repeats) locus of the insulin gene is associated with decreased body length, body weight, and head circumference at birth (21).
- Heterozygocity for a mutation in the glucokinase gene results in decreased birth weight (22).
- GLUT4 expression (only in muscle and fat, not liver) is impaired in young adults with insulin resistance who were undernourished in utero (23), which

- emphasizes the role of glucose transport in the control of insulin sensitivity
- suggests a mechanism for the relationship of insulin resistance and in utero undernutrition

ROLE OF MATERNAL DIABETES

- Assessment of fetal β-cell function by amniotic fluid insulin concentration (AFI) at 32–38 weeks gestation in 88 pregnancies with pregestational or gestational diabetes (24):
  - Offspring had annual oral glucose tolerance testing from age 18 months.
    - IGT was found in
      - 1.2% at <5 years of age
      - 5.4% at 5–9 years of age
      - 19.3% at 10–16 years of age
      - one-third of those with elevated AFI versus only 1 of 27 with normal AFI
    - There was no association between IGT and the type of maternal diabetes or the presence or absence of macrosomia at birth.
  - These results indicate the importance of the intrauterine environment as a risk factor for type 2 diabetes.
- The prevalence of diabetes in the offspring of Pima women with diabetes during pregnancy is significantly greater than that in
  - offspring of nondiabetic Pima women
  - offspring of women who later develop diabetes, emphasizing the important effect of diabetic pregnancy on altered β-cell function and glucoregulation later in life (25)
- The effect of maternal diabetes raises the specter of cumulative effects from generation to generation in increasing the prevalence of type 2 diabetes.

POLYCYSTIC OVARIAN SYNDROME AND PREMATURE ADRENARCHE

- There is increasing recognition of polycystic ovarian syndrome (PCOS) in the adolescent population (26).
- Girls with PCOS are reported to have ~40% reduction in insulin-stimulated glucose disposal compared with nonhyperandrogenic control subjects (27,28).

■ Premature adrenarche, which has been thought to be a benign condition, is now recognized as a risk factor for ovarian hyperandrogenism and PCOS (29).

■ Affected children are also more likely to have been born small for gestational age, indicating another aspect of the association of insulin resistance and intrauterine undernutrition (30,31).

RACIAL AND FAMILIAL INFLUENCES

■ Relative insulin resistance in African American compared with European American children:
  • In a biracial study of 377 subjects age 5–17 years, African American children had greater insulin responses to oral glucose than European American children, after adjustment for weight, age, obesity index, and pubertal stage (32).
  • In a biracial study of 1,200 subjects age 11–18 years (33), African American adolescents had higher insulin levels and lower glucose-to-insulin ratios than European American youths.
  • Prepubertal and pubertal African Americans have higher fasting and stimulated insulin concentrations during glucose clamp studies than European American youths (34).
  • Prepubertal African American children have lower C-peptide–to–insulin molar ratios than European American children, suggesting lower hepatic insulin clearance (35).
  • Rates of lipolysis are significantly lower in African American children than in European American children (36).
■ Relative energy conservation in African American vs. European American children, a phenotype that would be detrimental with nutritional surfeit (37):
  • Prepubertal African American children have lower maximum oxygen consumption during graded bicycle ergometry.
  • Prepubertal African American children have lower resting energy expenditure measured by indirect calorimetry after an overnight fast.
■ Family history of type 2 diabetes:
  • Family history is a risk factor for insulin resistance.
  • Prepubertal healthy African American children with a family history of type 2 diabetes ($n = 9$) and without such a history ($n = 13$) were studied (38).
    □ Subjects were matched for age, pubertal status, and total body adiposity, determined by dual-energy X-ray absorptiometry; abdominal obesity was determined by a computed tomography scan; and physi-

cal fitness was measured by maximum oxygen consumption with exercise.

□ A 3-hour hyperinsulinemic clamp study assessed insulin sensitivity.
□ Subjects with a family history of type 2 diabetes had lower insulin-stimulated glucose disposal and nonoxidative glucose disposal.

- BMI-matched children of Pima Indian parents with type 2 diabetes had decreased insulin sensitivity compared with children of parents who did not have diabetes (25).
- Familial clustering of type 2 diabetes also emphasizes the importance of environmental causation (39).
  □ Parents and siblings (n = 42) in 11 families of adolescents with type 2 diabetes were studied.
  □ Five mothers and 4 fathers had diabetes before the study. Diabetes was diagnosed in 3 additional fathers during the study.
  □ All 42 relatives had BMI >85th percentile and skinfold measurements >90th percentile.
  □ Fat intake was high and fiber intake low. Physical activity was nil to low.
  □ Eating disorders were common, and diabetes control was poor.

PUBERTY AND INSULIN RESISTANCE

- Physiological insulin resistance during puberty has been known for over 25 years (40).
- Mean age at diagnosis in all studies of type 2 diabetes in children is ~13.5 years, the peak time of pubertal growth and maturation (41).
- Insulin dose is substantially increased during puberty in patients with type 1 diabetes.
- Increased activity of the growth hormone–insulin-like growth factor (GH-IGF) axis is the likely explanation, because the insulin resistance is transitory and coincides with the time of maximal GH-IGF activity (42).

OBESITY AND INSULIN RESISTANCE:
THE ESSENTIAL PROBLEM

- Approximately 55% of the variance in insulin sensitivity in children matched for sex, age, ethnicity, and sexual maturation stage can be explained by total adiposity (43).
- Obese children have hyperinsulinism (which has been known for 30 years [44,45]) and an ~40% decrease in insulin-stimulated glucose metabolism compared to nonobese children (43) (Fig. 5).

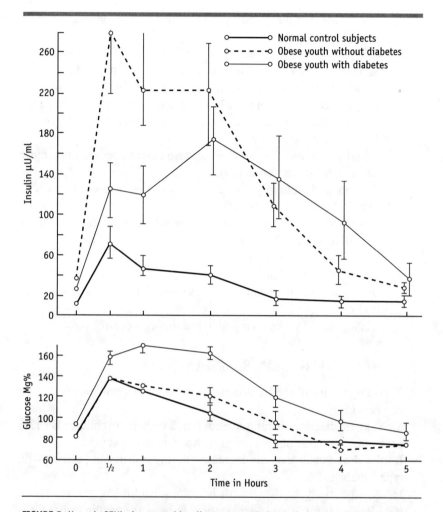

FIGURE 5. Mean (± SEM) glucose and insulin responses during oral glucose tolerance in normal weight pediatric control subjects, 7 obese youth with diabetes, and 11 obese youth without diabetes. Obese youth with normal glucose tolerance have approximately five times the insulin output of normal weight control subjects. Individuals with diabetes also have a severalfold greater insulin output, but it is inadequate to maintain normal glycemia in response to oral glucose. From Drash (44). Reprinted with permission from Elsevier Science.

- In a multiethnic study of 167 obese children and adolescents (46),
  - 25% of the children age 4–10 years and 21% of the adolescents age 11–18 years had IGT, and 4% of the adolescents had previously unrecognized diabetes
  - there was no evidence of insulin deficiency until decompensation

- African American children age 5–10 years ($n = 137$) had reduced insulin sensitivity, especially the girls, in proportion to increases in BP, triglycerides, subcutaneous fat, the percentage of total body fat, and Tanner stage of development (47).
- The amount of visceral fat in obese adolescents correlates directly with basal and glucose-stimulated insulinemia and inversely with insulin sensitivity and the rate of glucose uptake (48).
  - No correlation exists between subcutaneous fat and metabolic indexes.
  - These findings are similar to those in adults, indicating that even in the early stages of obesity, visceral fat is the most important determinant of glucose metabolism (49).
- Differences in metabolic effect of visceral fat as opposed to subcutaneous fat reflect the much greater lipolytic rate of visceral fat (Fig. 6).
- In a large study of ~9,500 German children age 5–6 years, the risk of overweight was markedly reduced by prolonged breast-feeding:
  - 3.8% of those who were exclusively breast-fed for 2 months versus 0.8% of those who were breast-fed for longer than 12 months became overweight (49).
  - Lower insulinemic responses are known to occur in breast-fed versus bottle-fed infants, and the former have lower energy and protein intake.
  - Association between early high protein intake and later adiposity has been described.

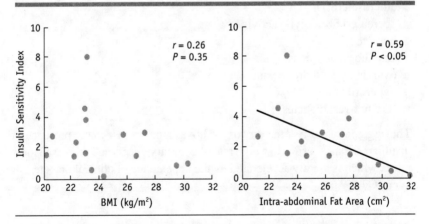

FIGURE 6. Insulin sensitivity relative to BMI and intra-abdominal fat. Insulin sensitivity index ($\times10^{-5}$ min^{-1}/pmol/l) in adults does not correlate with BMI but correlates strongly with intraabdominal fat area as measured by computed tomography scan. Adapted from Fujimoto et al. (49).

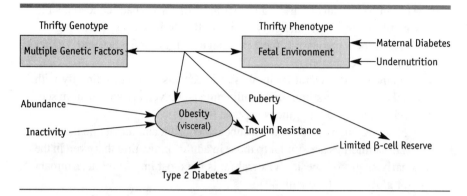

FIGURE 7. Factors in the development of type 2 diabetes.

THE INSULIN RESISTANCE SYNDROME (51)

Figure 7 summarizes the factors that have been discussed in the development of type 2 diabetes.

Diabetes is only one manifestation of the insulin resistance syndrome, a.k.a. the diabesity syndrome, syndrome X, or the metabolic syndrome, which includes (52)

- obesity as the core abnormality, specifically central (visceral) adiposity
- dyslipidemia
- atherosclerosis
- decreased fibrinolytic activity
- hypertension
- acanthosis nigricans
- ovarian hyperandrogenism
- hyperuricemia
- IGT to overt diabetes

The aggregation of risk factors for cardiovascular disease in the presence of insulin resistance results in a high rate of coronary events and increased mortality, which is greatly accelerated by the appearance of clinical diabetes, or even IGT (53).

Obesity

- In the large Bogalusa Heart Study (54) of the relationship of childhood obesity to coronary heart disease risk factors in adulthood

- 2,617 participants were examined at 2–17 years of age and reexamined at 18–37 years of age
- 77% of children with BMI ≥95th percentile remained obese as adults (BMI >30 kg/m^2)
- there were no differences in risk factors associated with obesity (hyperlipidemia, hypertension, or elevated insulin levels) among subjects who had been normal weight and subjects who had been overweight in childhood; thus, the increased risk of coronary heart disease related to childhood obesity is due to the persistence of the obesity in adulthood (54,55)

■ In addition to metabolic effects related to insulin resistance, obesity in childhood and adolescence has deleterious associations that increase morbidity or contribute to cardiovascular risk:

- elevated C-reactive protein and white blood cell counts, which have been associated with increased risk for cardiovascular disease in adults (56)
- proteinuria and focal segmental glomerular sclerosis in seven African American adolescents with severe obesity in the absence of diabetes (57)
- obstructive sleep apnea and other respiratory problems (58)
- hepatic steatosis (59)
- orthopedic problems (60)

Dyslipidemia (61)

■ Lipoprotein abnormalities in type 2 diabetes
- hypertriglyceridemia
- elevated very-low-density lipoprotein (VLDL) levels
- elevated LDL cholesterol
- elevated lipoprotein (a)
- decreased HDL cholesterol
- increased small, dense LDL particles
- decreased lipoprotein lipase activity
- increased lipoprotein glycation
- increased lipoprotein oxidation

■ Mechanism
- Fat cells that are sensitive to insulin store triglyceride and suppress hormone-sensitive lipase (the enzyme that breaks down triglycerides, releasing FFA).
- Insulin also provides glucose to fat cells for forming glycerol, the triglyceride backbone.

- Insulin resistance results in an abnormal breakdown of triglyceride stores and release of FFA and glycerol, contributing to gluconeogenesis.
  □ In muscle tissue, FFA cause insulin resistance.
  □ In liver, FFA are reconverted to triglyceride, driving the production of VLDL, the lipoprotein carrier of triglycerides, followed by other dyslipidemic changes.
- Hyperinsulinemia in the insulin-resistant state also drives the synthesis of fatty acids from glucose molecules in the liver.

Atherosclerosis (62)

- In adults, there is a strong association between the level of hyperglycemia and the increased risk of macrovascular disease.
- Dyslipidemia is one of several factors accelerating atherosclerosis in type 2 diabetes, including
  - oxidative stress
  - glycation of numerous vascular proteins
  - defective endothelium-dependent vasodilatation
  - elevated homocysteine
  - abnormalities of platelet function and coagulation
    □ increased fibrinogen
    □ increased plasminogen activator inhibitor 1
    □ decreased antithrombin III and other anticoagulation proteins (C & S)
    □ elevated Factors VII and VIII
    □ elevated vascular cell adhesion molecule 1
    □ increased platelet adhesiveness and aggregation
    □ decreased platelet nitric oxide production (nitric oxide mediates vasodilatation)
    □ decreased platelet prostacyclin production
    □ glycation of platelet proteins

Hypertension (63)

- Hypertension is estimated to account for 35–75% of diabetes complications, both microvascular and macrovascular (63).
- Diabetes or IGT doubles the risk of developing hypertension (64).
- Evidence is emerging of genetic predisposition to hypertension in type 2 diabetes related to the angiotensin-converting enzyme (ACE) genotype (65).
- Hypertension in type 2 diabetes is due to volume expansion and increased vascular resistance (62) related to

- reduced nitric oxide–mediated vasodilatation
- increased activity of the renin-angiotensin system

Acanthosis Nigricans

■ Acanthosis nigricans is considered a hallmark of insulin resistance and is a prominent feature of genetic insulin resistance syndromes not associated with obesity.

■ Acanthosis nigricans accompanying obesity in adolescents varies greatly by ethnicity, affecting ~90% of obese Native Americans, ~50% of obese African Americans, ~15% of obese Hispanic Americans, and <5% of obese European Americans (66).

■ As an indicator of hyperinsulinism, acanthosis nigricans also varies by ethnicity, inversely to its frequency of association with obesity (65).

■ Acanthosis nigricans is associated with IGT or type 2 diabetes in ~25% of individuals <20 years of age and in ~45% of those 20–30 years of age (65).

■ In a study of 139 overweight African American and European American children age 6–10 years (67)
- 50% of African Americans and 8.2% of European Americans had acanthosis nigricans
- half of the subjects with fasting hyperinsulinemia did not have acanthosis nigricans
- 80% of those with fasting hyperinsulinism had BMI ≥3 SD above normal for age and sex
- acanthosis nigricans was not a reliable marker for hyperinsulinemia in overweight children (although its presence in a child with diabetes was a diagnostic indicator)

REFERENCES

1. UKPDS Group: Intensive blood glucose control with sulphonylureas or insulin compared with conventional treatment and risk of complications in patients with type 2 diabetes (UKPDS 33). *Lancet* 352:837–853, 1998
2. Neel JV: Diabetes mellitus: a "thrifty" genotype rendered detrimental by "progress"? *Am J Hum Genet* 14:353–362, 1962
3. Lev-Ran A: Thrifty genotype: how applicable is it to obesity and type 2 diabetes? *Diabetes Reviews* 7:1–22, 1999
4. Lindgren CM, Hirschhorn JN: The genetics of type 2 diabetes. *Endocrinologist* 11:178–187, 2001
5. Rosenbloom AL, Joe JR, Young RS, Winter WE: The emerging epidemic of type 2 diabetes mellitus in youth. *Diabetes Care* 22:345–354, 1999

6. Winter WE, Nakamura M, House DV: Monogenic diabetes mellitus in youth: the MODY syndromes. *Endocrinol Metab Clin North Am* 28:765–785, 1999
7. Rosenbloom AL, House DV, Winter WE: Non-insulin dependent diabetes mellitus (NIDDM) in minority youth: research priorities and needs. *Clin Pediatr* 37:143–152, 1998
8. Hanis CL, Boerwinkle E, Chakraborty R, Ellsworth DL, Concannon P, Stirling B, et al.: A genome-wide search for human non-insulin-dependent (type 2) diabetes genes reveals a major susceptibility locus on chromosome 2. *Nat Genet* 13:161–166, 1996
9. Horikawa Y, Oda N, Cox NJ, Li X, Orho-Melander M, Hara M, et al.: Genetic variation in the gene encoding calpain-10 is associated with type 2 diabetes mellitus. *Nat Genet* 26:163–175, 2000
10. Baier LJ, Permana PA, Yang X, Pratley RE, Hanson RL, Shen GQ, et al.: A calpain-10 gene polymorphism is associated with reduced muscle mRNA levels and insulin resistance. *J Clin Invest* 106:R69–R73, 2000
11. Phipps K, Barker DJP: Fetal growth and impaired glucose tolerance in men and women. *Diabetologia* 36:225–228, 1993
12. Phillips DI, Barker DJ, Hales CN, Hirst S, Osmond C: Thinness at birth and insulin resistance in adult life. *Diabetologia* 37:150–154, 1994
13. Lithell HO, McKeigue PM, Berglund L, Mohsen R, Lithell UB, Leon DA: Relation at birth to non-insulin-dependent diabetes and insulin concentrations in men aged 50-60 years. *BMJ* 312:406–410, 1996
14. Curhan GC, Willett WC, Rimm EB, Spiegelman D, Ascherio AL, Stampfer MJ: Birth weight and adult hypertension, diabetes mellitus, and obesity in US men. *Circulation* 94:3246–3250, 1996
15. Dabelea D, Pettitt DJ, Hanson RL, Imperatore G, Bennett PH, Knowler WC: Birth weight, type 2 diabetes, and insulin resistance in Pima Indian children and young adults. *Diabetes Care* 22:944–950, 1999
16. Montgomery SM, Ekbom A: Smoking during pregnancy and diabetes mellitus in a British longitudinal birth cohort. *BMJ* 321:26–27, 2002
17. Jaquett D, Gaboriau A, Czernichow P, Levy-Marchal C: Insulin resistance early in adulthood in subjects born with intrauterine growth retardation. *J Clin Endocrinol Metab* 85:1401–1406, 2000
18. Bavdekar A, Yajnik CS, Fall CH, Bapat S, Pandit AN, Deshpande V, et al.: Insulin resistance syndrome in 8-year-old Indian children: small at birth, big at 8 years, or both? *Diabetes* 48:2422–2429, 1999
19. Li C, Johnson MS, Goran MI: Effects of low birth weight on insulin resistance syndrome in Caucasian and African-American children. *Diabetes Care* 24:2035–2042, 2001
20. Wei JN, Sung FC, Li CY, Chang CH, Lin RS, Lin CC, Chiang CC, Chuang LM: Low birth weight and high birth weight infants are both at an increased risk to have type 2 diabetes among schoolchildren in Taiwan. *Diabetes Care* 26:343–348, 2003
21. Dunger DB, Ong KK, Huxtable SJ, Sherriff A, Woods KA, Ahmed ML, et al.: Association of the INS VNTR with size at birth: ALSPAC Study Team: Avon Longitudinal Study of Pregnancy and Childhood. *Nat Genet* 19:98–100, 1998

22. Hattersley AT, Beards F, Ballantyne E, Appleton M, Harvey R, Ellard S: Mutations in the glucokinase gene of the fetus result in reduced birth weight. *Nat Genet* 19:268–270, 1998

23. Jaquett D, Vidal H, Hankard R, Czernichow P, Levy-Marchal C: Impaired regulation of glucose transporter 4 gene expression in insulin resistance associated with in utero undernutrition. *J Clin Endocrinol Metab* 86:3266–3271, 2001

24. Silverman BL, Metzger BE, Cho NH, Loeb CA: Impaired glucose tolerance in adolescent offspring of diabetic mothers: relationship to fetal hyperinsulinism. *Diabetes Care* 18:611–617, 1995

25. Pettitt DJ, Aleck KA, Baird HR, Carraher MJ, Bennett PH, Knowler WC: Congenital susceptibility to NIDDM: Role of intrauterine environment. *Diabetes* 37:622–628, 1988

26. Legro RS, Kunselman AR, Dodson WC, Dunaif A: Prevalence and predictors of risk for type 2 diabetes mellitus and impaired glucose tolerance in polycystic ovary syndrome: a prospective, controlled study in 254 affected women. *J Clin Endocrinol Metab* 84:165–169, 1999

27. Lewy V, Danadian K, Arslanian SA: Early metabolic abnormalities in adolescents with polycystic ovarian syndrome (PCOS). *Pediatr Res* 45:93A, 1999

28. Lewy V, Danadian K, Arslanian SA: Roles of insulin resistance and β-cell dysfunction in the pathogenesis of glucose intolerance in adolescents with polycystic ovary syndrome (Abstract). *Diabetes* 48:A292, 1999

29. Banerjee S, Raghavan S, Wasserman EJ, Linder BL, Saenger P, DiMartino-Nardi J: Hormonal findings in African-American and Caribbean Hispanic girls with premature adrenarche: implications for polycystic ovarian syndrome. *Pediatrics* 102:E36, 1998

30. Vuguin P, Linder B, Rosenfeld RG, Saenger P, DiMartino-Nardi J: The roles of insulin sensitivity, insulin-like growth factor I (IGF-I), and IGF-binding protein-1 and -3 in the hyperandrogenism of African-American and Caribbean Hispanic girls with premature adrenarche. *J Clin Endocrinol Metab* 84:2037–2042, 1999

31. Ibañez L, Potau N, Marcos MV, deZegher F: Exaggerated adrenarche and hyperinsulinism in adolescent girls born small for gestational age. *J Clin Endocrinol Metab* 84:4739–4741, 1999

32. Svec F, Nastasi K, Hilton C, Bao W, Srinivasan SR, Berenson GS: Black-white contrasts and insulin levels during pubertal development: the Bogalusa Heart Study. *Diabetes* 41:313–317, 1992

33. Jiang X, Srinivasan SR, Radhakrishnamurthy B, Dalferes ER, Berenson GS: Racial (black-white) differences in insulin secretion and clearance in adolescents: the Bogalusa heart study. *Pediatrics* 97:357–360, 1996

34. Arslanian S: Insulin secretion and sensitivity in healthy African-American vs. American-white children. *Clin Pediatr* 37:81–88, 1998

35. Uwaife GI, Nguyen TT, Keil MF, Russell DL, Nicholson JC, Bonat SH, et al.: Differences in insulin secretion and sensitivity of Caucasian and African-American prepubertal children. *J Pediatr* 140:673–680, 2002

36. Danadian K, Lewy V, Janosky JJ, Arslanian S: Lipolysis in African-American children: is it a metabolic risk factor predisposing to obesity? *J Clin Endocrinol Metab* 86:3022–3026, 2001

37. Kaplan AS, Zernel BS, Stallings VA: Differences in resting energy expenditure in prepubertal black children and white children. *J Pediatr* 129:643–647, 1996
38. Danadian K, Balasekaran G, Lewy V, Meza MP, Robertson R, Arslanian SA: Insulin sensitivity in African-American children with and without a family history of type 2 diabetes. *Diabetes Care* 22:1325–1329, 1999
39. Pinhas-Hamiel O, Standiford D, Hamiel D, Dolan LM, Cohen R, Zeitler PS: The type 2 family: a setting for development and treatment of adolescent type 2 diabetes mellitus. *Arch Pediatr Adolesc Med* 153:1063–1067, 1999
40. Rosenbloom AL, Wheeler L, Bianchi R, Chin FT, Tiwary CM, Grgic A: Age adjusted analysis of insulin responses during normal and abnormal oral glucose tolerance tests in children and adolescents. *Diabetes* 24:820–828, 1975
41. Fagot-Campagna A, Pettitt DJ, Engelgau MM, Burrows NR, Geiss LS, Valdez R, et al.: Type 2 diabetes among North American children and adolescents: an epidemiological review and a public health perspective. *J Pediat* 136:664–672, 2000
42. American Diabetes Association: Type 2 diabetes in children and adolescents (Consensus Statement) *Diabetes Care* 23:381–389, 2000
43. Caprio S, Tamborlane WV: Metabolic impact of obesity in childhood. *Metab Clin North Am* 28:731–747, 1999
44. Drash AM: Relationship between diabetes mellitus and obesity in the child. *Metabolism* 22:337–344, 1973
45. Martin MM, Martin AL: Obesity, hyperinsulinism, and diabetes mellitus in childhood. *J Pediatr* 82:192–201, 1973
46. Sinha R, Fisch G, Teague B, Tamborlane WV, Banyas B, Allen K, et al.: Prevalence of impaired glucose tolerance among children and adolescents with marked obesity. *N Engl J Med* 346:802–810, 2002
47. Young-Hyman D, Schlundt DG, Herman L, DeLuca F, Counts D: Evaluation of the insulin resistance syndrome in 5- to 10-year-old overweight/obese African-American children. *Diabetes Care* 24:1359–1364, 2001
48. Caprio S: Relationship between abdominal visceral fat and metabolic risk factors in obese adolescents. *Am J Hum Biol* 11:259–266, 1999
49. Fujimoto WY, Abbate SL, Kahn SE, Hokanson JE, Brunzell JD: The visceral adiposity syndrome in Japanese-American men. *Obes Res* 2:364–371, 1994
50. von Kries R, Koletzko B, Sauerwald T, von Mutius E, Barnert D, Grunert V, et al.: Breast feeding and obesity: cross sectional study. *BMJ* 319:147–150, 1999
51. Rosenbloom AL: What is the cause of the epidemic of type 2 diabetes in children? *Curr Opin Endocrinol Diabetes* 7:191–196, 2000
52. American Diabetes Association: Consensus Development Conference On Insulin Resistance: 5–6 November 1997. *Diabetes Care* 21:310–314, 1998
53. Expert Committee on the Diagnosis and Classification of Diabetes Mellitus: Report of the Expert Committee on the Diagnosis and Classification of Diabetes Mellitus. *Diabetes Care* 24 (Suppl. 1):S5–S20, 2001
54. Freedman DS, Khan LK, Dietz WH, Srinivasan SR, Berenson GS: Relationship of childhood obesity to coronary heart disease risk factors in adulthood: the Bogalusa Heart Study. *J Pediatr* 108:712–718, 2001

55. Steinberger J, Moran A, Hong C-P, Jacobs DR, Sinaiko AR: Adiposity in childhood predicts obesity and insulin resistance in young adulthood. *J Pediatr* 138:469–473, 2001

56. Visser M, Bouter LM, McQuillan GM, Wener MH, Harris TB: Low grade systemic inflammation in overweight children. *Pediatrics* 107:E13, 2001

57. Adelman RD, Restaino IG, Alon US, Blowey DL: Proteinurea and focal segmental glomerulosclerosis in severely obese adolescents. *J Pediatr* 138:481–485, 2001

58. de la Eva RC, Bauer LA, Donahue KC, Waters KA: Metabolic correlates with obstructive sleep apnea in obese subjects. *J Pediatr* 140:654–659, 2002

59. Strauss RS, Barlow SE, Dietz WH: Prevalence of abnormal serum aminotransferase values in overweight and obese adolescents. *J Pediatr* 136:727–733, 2000

60. Smith JC, Field C, Braden DS, Gaymes CH, Kastner J: Coexisting health problems in obese children and adolescents that might require special treatment considerations. *Clin Pediatr* 38:305–307, 1999

61. Goldberg IJ: Diabetic dyslipidemia: causes and consequences. *J Clin Endocrinol Metab* 86:965–971, 2001

62. Kirpichnikov D, Sowers JR: Diabetes mellitus and diabetes-associated vascular disease. *Trends Endocrinol Metab* 12:225–230, 2001

63. Gress TW, Nieto FJ, Shahar E, Wofford MR, Brancati FL: Hypertension and antihypertensive therapy as risk factors for type 2 diabetes mellitus: Atherosclerosis Risk in Community Study. *N Engl J Med* 342:905–912, 2000

64. Salomaa VV, Strandberg TE, Vanhanen H, Naukkarinen V, Sarna S, Miettinen TA: Glucose tolerance and blood pressure: long-term follow-up in middle-age men. *BMJ* 302:493–496, 1991

65. Wierzbicki AS, Nimmo L, Feher MD, Cox A, Foxton J, Lant AF: Association of angiotensin-converting enzyme DD genotype with hypertension in diabetes. *J Hum Hypertens* 9:671–673, 1995

66. Stuart CA, Gilkison CR, Smith MM, Bosma AM, Keenan BS, Nagamani M: Acanthosis nigricans as a risk factor for noninsulin dependent diabetes mellitus. *Clin Pediatr* 37:73–80, 1998

67. Nguyen TT, Keil MF, Russell DL, Pathomvanich A, Uwaifo GI, Sebring NG, et al.: Relation of acanthosis nigricans to hyperinsulinemia and insulin sensitivity in overweight African-American and white children. *J Pediatr* 138:474–480, 2001

CHAPTER 5

Case Finding: Who Should Be Tested?

EPIDEMIOLOGIC CRITERIA FOR CASE FINDING

Case finding is the appropriate description for type 2 diabetes testing in obese children and refers to diagnostic testing in an at-risk population (1). In this situation, the screening test was the determination of obesity.

■ Justification for case finding (2):
- **The condition tested for is sufficiently common to justify the investment.** Type 2 diabetes is sufficiently common in obese children and youth to justify testing them, especially those with other features of insulin resistance, high-risk ethnicity, or family history of type 2 diabetes.
- **The condition tested for is serious in terms of morbidity and mortality.** This is unquestionably true of type 2 diabetes in children because of the association with increased cardiovascular risk factors.
- **The condition tested for has a prolonged latency period without symptoms, during which abnormality can be detected.** Type 2 diabetes in children is often detected in the asymptomatic state, but albuminuria and dyslipidemia may already be present, indicating a prolonged latency period, as in adults.
- **A test is available that is sensitive (few false-negative results) and accurate, with acceptable specificity (minimal number of false-positive results).** The fasting plasma glucose and 2-hour plasma glucose have been applied to high-risk populations and are exceptionally sensitive and specific. Random opportunistic glucose measurements may be appropriate and are likely to be sensitive.

- **An intervention is available to prevent or delay disease onset or more effectively treat the condition detected in the latency phase.** The societal, family, community, and personal resources needed to prevent or delay the development of serious manifestations of the insulin resistance syndrome present a daunting challenge.

TESTING RECOMMENDATIONS

The consensus panel of the ADA (3) made the recommendations outlined in Table 12.

- If necessary for convenience, glucose can be measured in patients who have had food shortly before testing, with a random plasma glucose concentration of ≥140 mg/dl (7.8 mmol/l), an indication for further testing (3).
- These criteria were established without a database and therefore should not replace individual clinical judgment, as recognized by the consensus panel (3).
- Although fasting plasma glucose was deemed preferable because of lower cost and greater convenience, considerable sensitivity may be lost because the 2-hour plasma glucose usually increases earlier than the fasting glucose in the course of development of type 2 diabetes (4).

TABLE 12. Testing for Type 2 Diabetes in Children

Criteria*: Overweight >BMI (85th percentile for age and sex [Figs. 8 and 9], weight for height >85th percentile, or weight >120% of ideal for height)

PLUS

Any two of the following risk factors:

- Family history of type 2 diabetes in first- or second-degree relative
- High-risk race/ethnicity (American Indian, African American, Hispanic, or Asian/Pacific Islander)
- Signs of insulin resistance or conditions associated with insulin resistance (acanthosis nigricans, hypertension, dyslipidemia, or PCOS)

⇒ **Age of initiation:** Age 10 years or at onset of puberty, if puberty occurs at a younger age
⇒ **Frequency:** Every 2 years
⇒ **Test:** Fasting plasma glucose preferred

*Clinical judgment should be used to test for diabetes in high-risk patients who do not meet these criteria.

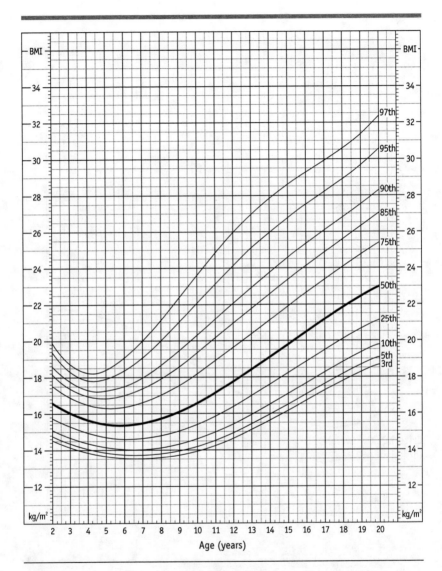

FIGURE 8. BMI percentiles for age in boys 2–20 years of age. Source: Developed by the National Center for Health Statistics in collaboration with the National Center for Chronic Disease Prevention and Health Promotion (2000).

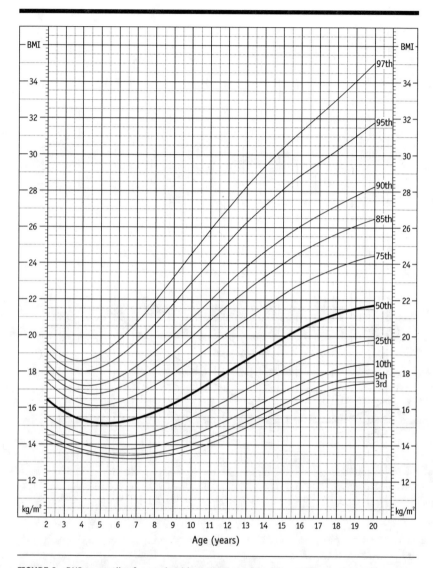

FIGURE 9. BMI percentiles for age in girls 2–20 years of age. Source: Developed by the National Center for Health Statistics in collaboration with the National Center for Chronic Disease Prevention and Health Promotion (2000).

- Cellular glucose uptake is largely (~75%) insulin independent (central nervous system 50%, splanchnic organs 25%) during the fasting state, when insulin levels are low.
- Thus, insulin resistance peripherally has little effect on fasting glucose, which will increase when insulin deficiency has progressed to the point of increasing fasting hepatic glucose production (5).
- In obese adults, fasting plasma glucose was found to be highly insensitive compared with oral glucose tolerance testing for the detection of diabetes (6).

■ Although type 2 diabetes is disproportionately seen in both adults and children from certain ethnic/racial groups, substantial numbers of white, non-Hispanic children, adolescents, and adults are also affected, making high-risk ethnicity an insensitive criterion for testing. A recent report on the testing of a multiethnic cohort of 167 severely obese children and adolescents found IGT and silent type 2 diabetes in substantial numbers regardless of ethnicity (7). Outside of North America, South Asian and Middle Eastern populations are also disproportionately at risk (see Chapter 3).

■ The age suggested in the criteria may be too limiting, particularly with increasing numbers of obese youth under 10 years of age being seen with type 2 diabetes and pre-diabetes. The study noted above found that 25% of the 55 obese children age 4–10 years had IGT, as did 21% of the 112 adolescents age 11–18 years (6).

REFERENCES

1. Fletcher RH, Fletcher SW, Wagner EH: *Clinical Epidemiology: the Essentials.* 2nd ed. Baltimore, MD, Williams and Wilkins, 1988
2. Sackett DL, Holland WW: Controversy in detection of disease. *Lancet* 2:357–359, 1965
3. American Diabetes Association. Type 2 diabetes in children and adolescents (Consensus Statement). *Diabetes Care* 23:381–389, 2000
4. DeFronzo RA: Lilly Lecture. The triumvirate: beta cell, muscle, liver: a collusion responsible for NIDDM. *Diabetes* 37:667–687, 1998
5. Ferrannini E, DeFronzo RA: Insulin actions *in vivo:* glucose metabolism. In *International Textbook of Diabetes Mellitus.* 2nd ed. Alberti KGMM, Zimmet P, DeFronzo RA, Keen H, Eds. Chichester, U.K., Wiley, 1997, p. 503–530
6. Richard JL, Sultan A, Daures J-P, Vannereau D, Parer-Richard C: Diagnosis of diabetes mellitus and intermediate glucose abnormalities in obese patients based on ADA (1997) and WHO (1985) criteria. *Diabet Med* 19:292–299, 2002
7. Sinha R, Fisch G, Teague B, Tamborlane WV, Banyas B, Allen K, et al.: Prevalence of impaired glucose tolerance among children and adolescents with marked obesity. *N Engl J Med* 346:802–810, 2002

Is Type 2 Diabetes in Children Preventable? The Individual and Community Challenge

DEFINITIONS (1)

Primary Prevention/Intervention

- intervention preventing or delaying the development of disease (e.g., obesity) in individuals identified as high risk
- intervention directed at populations at risk

Secondary Prevention/Intervention

- treatment of individuals who have developed a disease to prevent or delay the development of complications (e.g., the insulin resistance syndrome)
- population-directed programs of awareness and education for instigation and support of intervention

Tertiary Prevention/Intervention

- intervention to minimize or reverse the deleterious effects of complications
- treatment of type 2 diabetes and other comorbidities of the insulin resistance syndrome

This chapter will consider primary and secondary prevention; treatment of type 2 diabetes and its complications (tertiary intervention) will be discussed in Chapter 7.

PRIMARY PREVENTION/INTERVENTION

Justification for Intervention in Childhood

- The epidemic of obesity and its complications account for a substantial and increasing proportion of direct and indirect health care costs (2–7).
- Obesity is associated with diminished school performance because of sleep apnea, torpor associated with lack of physical exercise, and social stigmatization.
- The high frequency of obesity and its comorbidities in young men and women reduces the pool of able-bodied individuals for civil and military duty, making primary prevention a strategic necessity for the nation.
- Secondary prevention of obesity is rarely successful beyond the short term.
- Intervention in adult populations, exemplified by the 13-year Minnesota Heart Health Program involving six communities, reflects the difficulty in altering lifestyle and dietary habits (8).
  - Adult education classes provided training for weight control, exercise, and cholesterol reduction.
  - Workplace weight control programs, home correspondence courses, and weight gain prevention programs were offered.
  - There was a strong upward trend in weight, even when considering potential confounding variables.

Problems in Implementation

- challenge of countering eating and entertainment trends that provide popular social outlets and are highly attractive, ubiquitous, and heavily promoted
- incentives for financially stressed school systems to provide fast-food concessions and soft drink and snack vending machines
- alternative food lines in middle schools and high schools serving high-fat, high-calorie foods such as pizza and French fries
- decline in compulsory physical education programs in schools and lack of noncompetitive programs permitting participation of all students (e.g., aerobics, dance)

- lack of safe environments for regular physical activity in some communities
- failure to recognize childhood obesity as an avoidable disease state
- lack of funding for after-school programs, including transportation support
- school curricula that do not address obesity prevention, or without plans for incorporating healthy lifestyle training into traditional curricula
- need for commitment of the community and of the family which is frequently disorganized for such an endeavor

Approaches

- School-based behavior interventions
  - Planet Health (1,295 boys and girls in grades 6–8 [9]):
    - □ 2 school years of sessions to encourage decreased television viewing and consumption of high-fat foods, increased fruit and vegetable intake, and increased moderate and vigorous physical activity
    - □ prevalence of obesity among participating girls reduced compared with control subjects
  - Child and Adolescent Trial for Cardiovascular Health (CATCH) (10):
    - □ Texas program to train teachers and food service staff, based on National Heart Lung and Blood Institute program, authorized by the Texas legislature in 1999
    - □ teaches primary school students elements of a healthy diet and a physically active lifestyle, promoting lower-fat and lower-sodium foods, regular exercise, and avoidance of tobacco products
    - □ school lunches that average no more than 30% of calories from fat
    - □ 50% of physical education class time spent in vigorous physical activity
  - Bienestar Health Program (11):
    - □ 4th grade Mexican American children
    - □ program based on social cognitive theory, social system structure, and culturally relevant material
    - □ learning activities developed for social systems influencing the children's health behaviors, such as parents, the classroom, the school cafeteria, and after-school care
    - □ initial results (first 2 years of the program):
      - ○ significant decrease in dietary fat servings and the percentage of total calories from fat; significant increase of dietary fruit and vegetable servings and of diabetes health knowledge

○ no decrease in percentage of body fat, and no increase in level of physical activity
- Quest program (12), begun in 1996 for Pima elementary schoolchildren (K–2):
  □ biochemical and anthropometric monitoring
  □ classroom instruction about diabetes
  □ increased daily physical activity at school
  □ structured school breakfast and lunch programs with rewards for the school for adherence
- Eat Well and Keep Moving Program (13):
  □ interdisciplinary health behavior intervention for children in grades 4 and 5 in six intervention and eight matched control schools, involving 479 students
  □ classroom curriculum for teachers of math, science, language arts, and social studies over a 2-year period
  □ links to school food services and families, with training and wellness programs for teachers and other staff members
  □ results: reduction in total energy from fat and saturated fat, an increase in fruit and vegetable intake, and a slight reduction in television viewing
- Kahnawake Schools Diabetes Prevention Project (14):
  □ behavioral change theory with a health promotion planning model and native learning styles
  □ focused on elementary schoolchildren
  □ 87% of experimental and 71% of comparison school parents consented
- Trial (randomized, controlled) of reducing television, videotape, and videogame use by 3rd and 4th grade students (~200) (15):
  □ 18-lesson, 6-month classroom curriculum
  □ significant reduction in relative BMI
  □ significant decrease in television viewing and meals eaten in front of the television
  □ no changes in high-fat food intake, moderate to vigorous physical activity, or cardiorespiratory fitness
- SPARK program (www.foundation.sdsu.edu/projects/spark), Florida experience:
  □ after-school intervention involving brief nutrition education integrated with staged, age-appropriate exercise skills for elementary schoolchildren over 2 years
  □ results at 1 year:

- ○ more free time spent playing outdoors, practicing newly learned skills
- ○ decreased resting heart rate in 4th and 5th grade children
- ○ no difference in BMI between intervention ($n = 73$) and control ($n = 89$) groups
- ■ Community-based Zuni Diabetes Prevention Program (16):
  - ● designed to reduce diabetes risk factors in Zuni Indian high school youth
  - ● intervention strategies:
    - □ supportive social networks (parent-teacher organizations, faculty groups, and paid youth) developing assessment databases and leadership
    - □ development of a wellness facility outfitted with workout equipment and serving as a base for vigorous outings
    - □ integrated diabetes education incorporating relevant material into home economics/food service, biology, geometry, and computer science
    - □ modification of the food supply (eliminating sugar-containing beverages from the vending machines in the school; identifying and eliminating barriers to healthy food in the school cafeteria)
  - ● 2-year results:
    - □ reduction in BMI, decreased consumption of sugar-containing beverages, increased dietary fiber, decreased sitting pulse rates, and increased glucose-to-insulin ratios
    - □ changes only in beverage consumption and insulin levels significant
- ■ Family and individual intervention:
  - ● Prolonged breast-feeding reduces the risk of obesity in childhood (17).
  - ● Children with normal-weight parents have a <7% risk of becoming overweight, whereas those with one overweight parent have a 40% risk and those with both parents overweight have an 80% risk (18).
  - ● Parent training by pediatricians, WIC (Women, Infants, and Children Program) nurses, and other health care personnel should emphasize several basic concepts.
    - □ A fat baby is not a healthier baby.
    - □ Candy, potato chips, and other poorly nutritious food should not be used as a reward.
    - □ An obesity-preventing diet is important for the entire family and will not work for any one family member alone.

□ Similarly, physical activity needs to be promoted as a family. This activity need not be organized, but it should involve daily efforts to be physically more active, such as using stairs instead of elevators, walking or bicycling to school or to work, and doing house and yard work.
□ Restricting television viewing will result in increased physical activity.
□ Meals should be taken on schedule, in one place, with no other activity (television, studying, reading, or playing).

SECONDARY PREVENTION/INTERVENTION

The prevention of diabetes and other complications of insulin resistance in overweight children and adolescents is as daunting as it is important for individual and public health. The primary prevention efforts in schools and communities will be secondary prevention initiatives for the substantial and variable proportion of youths who are already overweight. For these youths, further considerations include:

- behavioral modification: eating and exercise
- medications: appetite reducing, nutrient absorption blocking, or thermogenesis enhancing
- surgery: gastric bypass, flexible banding, or stapling

Behavior Modification in Pre-diabetes

- Individuals with impaired fasting glucose, defined by a glucose level 110–126 mg/dl, and IGT (2-hour postprandial blood glucose level of 140–200 mg/dl) are considered to have pre-diabetes.
- Studies in adults indicate that lifestyle interventions improve glucose tolerance in individuals at high risk for developing type 2 diabetes, at least over the short term.
  - Da Qing IGT and Diabetes Study (19):
    □ six year study of Chinese men with IGT randomized to dietary and exercise intervention ($n = 126$) or a control nonintervention group ($n = 133$)
    □ type 2 diabetes 32% less frequent with intervention
  - Finnish Diabetes Prevention Study (20):
    □ 522 middle-aged overweight subjects (172 men), mean age 55 years, mean BMI 31 kg/m^2, all with IGT
    □ randomized to a control group or an intervention group
    □ individualized counseling to reduce weight (subjects met with a nutritionist seven times the 1st year and every 3 months thereafter),

reduce total and saturated fat intake, and increase fiber intake and exercise
- annual oral glucose tolerance test; mean follow-up 3.2 years
- moderate weight loss, and >50% reduction in progression to diabetes (11 vs. 23% in control subjects)
- Australian reduced-fat diet intervention study (21):
  - 136 adults with pre-diabetes recruited from the Workforce Diabetes Survey
  - subjects randomized to a control group or an intervention group (reduced-fat diet reinforced by monthly small-group education sessions for 1 year)
  - groups followed for 5 years
  - modest weight loss in the intervention group sustained for 2 years but not for 5 years
  - at end of the first year, fewer in the intervention group with diabetes or pre-diabetes (47%) than in the control group (67%); no differences thereafter
  - more compliant 50% of the intervention group with sustained lower fasting and 2-hour glucose levels at 5 years
- The Diabetes Prevention Program (22):
  - study of 3,234 adults (mean age 51 years) with risk factors of obesity (mean BMI 34 kg/m^2) and elevated but not diabetic fasting and post-load plasma glucose concentrations
  - subjects randomly assigned to placebo or metformin (850 mg twice daily) with usual diet and exercise counseling or intensive lifestyle modification (at least 7% weight loss in a week and at least 150 minutes physical activity per week)
  - intensive group able to maintain a 5% weight loss over a 3-year period, with 14% developing diabetes compared with 22% in the metformin group and 29% in the placebo group
  - estimated that to prevent one case of diabetes over a 3-year period, 7 people would have to participate in the lifestyle intervention and 14 would have to receive metformin
- Children, especially preadolescents, are more likely to maintain weight control than adults (23).
  - Five- and 10-year results indicate successful maintenance by a substantial portion of subjects.
  - In 113 treated families using family-based intervention, children had greater relative weight loss and better maintenance than adults, with one-third of children being nonobese after 10 years.

- Study of 24 families, including children 8–12 years old, participating in a 10- to 12-session behavioral intervention (24):
  - □ Two-thirds of families completed the treatment program.
  - □ Children who completed the program lost weight.
  - □ Weight loss was not maintained during 4–13 months of follow-up.
- Even the modest successes in reported studies must be tempered by the realization that these are select study populations.
- General intervention principles:
  - Begin as early as possible.
  - Co-opt the family, who must be committed to change and participation.
  - The family and older child should understand the medical implications of obesity.
  - Make changes in small increments and with the understanding that these are permanent lifestyle changes.
  - Train the patient and family in monitoring quantity and quality of food, eating behavior, and physical activity.
  - Recognize that there is a high rate of depression (>50%) in overweight adolescents.
  - Encourage, positively reinforce, and commend minor achievement (e.g., no or minimal weight gain with gain in height or reduction in high-caloric drinks) and empathize with setbacks.
  - Educate parents for healthy behavior reinforcement.
    - □ Encourage and praise physical activity (yard work, stairs instead of elevators, etc.).
    - □ Limit television.
    - □ Do not use food as a reward.
    - □ Have meals at regular times without distractions (television, homework, videogames, etc.). Control portions.
    - □ Do not stock the pantry and refrigerator with high-fat, calorically dense food and drink. Read labels and control purchasing.
    - □ Serve as a role model in avoiding gastronomic temptation and enjoying healthy eating and physical exercise.

Medication (7,25)

No medications are currently approved for use in children to treat obesity. Long-term studies in adults indicate that cessation of medication is followed by the regain of lost weight.

- Orlistat
  - inhibits pancreatic lipase, decreasing intestinal fat absorption by ~30%
  - improves lipidemia and glycemia in adults
  - causes weight loss if there is not increased intake of nonfat calories
  - no published studies in children
- Sibutramine
  - reuptake inhibitor of serotonin and norepinephrine
  - increases satiety with a minimal effect on appetite
  - stimulates fasting and postprandial thermogenesis
  - no published studies in children
- Buproprion HCl
  - antidepressant chemically unrelated to tricyclic, heterocyclic, selective serotonin reuptake inhibitor, or other known agents
  - use associated with appetite suppression
- Other drugs frequently found in over-the-counter weight loss preparations: caffeine, ephedrine, and ephedra
  - ephedrine/caffeine combination with caloric restriction more effective than diet alone in a controlled study in adults
  - no published studies in children; potential side effects make studies unlikely
- Metformin
  - only drug studied in at-risk children (26)
  - 29 Caucasian and African American adolescents 12–19 years old with BMI >30 kg/m^2
  - enrollment with elevated fasting insulin (>15 μU/ml), first- or second-degree relative with type 2 diabetes, and normal fasting glucose levels and A1C
  - metformin (500 mg b.i.d.) or placebo for 6 months
  - BMI mean rise of 0.23 SD in control and decrease of 0.12 SD in metformin-treated subjects ($P < 0.02$)
  - decreased fasting glucose ($P < 0.02$) and insulin levels ($P < 0.01$) with metformin
  - transient abdominal discomfort or diarrhea in 40% of metformin-treated subjects

Surgery (27)

- The National Institutes of Health Clinical Guidelines on the Identification, Evaluation, and Treatment of Overweight and Obesity in Adults indicate that gastric bypass surgery is appropriate for select adults with BMI ≥40 or ≥35 kg/m² with comorbidity.

■ Limited data and no guidelines exist for children and adolescents.

■ In a 1975 report, median weight loss was ~25% 3 years after gastric bypass or gastroplasty in 18 morbidly obese adolescents.

■ In a 1980 report, average weight loss was 40 kg at 3 years and 26 kg at 5 years after gastric bypass or gastroplasty in 30 patients <20 years of age. Major postoperative complications in one-third of patients included one postoperative death from anastomosis leak.

■ In a 2001 report, 10 adolescents ≤17 years of age who had gastric bypass surgery with newer techniques (28):
  ● follow-up >1 year in 9 subjects
  ● no postoperative complications
  ● resolution of obesity-related morbidities in 7 patients (sleep apnea, hypertension, dyspnea, vertebral compression fracture, refusal to attend school)
  ● >30-kg weight loss in nine patients
  ● late complications requiring surgery in 4 patients (incisional hernia, cholecystectomy, small bowel obstruction).
  ● medical complications: mild iron deficiency anemia and transient folate deficiency

REFERENCES

1. Fletcher RH, Fletcher SW, Wagner EH: *Clinical Epidemiology: The Essentials.* 2nd ed. Baltimore, MD, Williams and Wilkins, 1988
2. Sokol RJ: The chronic disease of childhood obesity: the sleeping giant has awakened. *J Pediatr* 136:711–713, 2000
3. Tersbakovec AM, Watson MH, Wenner WJ, Marx AL: Insurance reimbursement for treatment of obesity in children. *J Pediatr* 134:573–578, 1999
4. Zwiaur KFM: Prevention and treatment of overweight and obesity in children and adolescents. *Eur J Pediatr* 159 (Suppl. 1):S56–S68, 2000
5. Segel DG, Sanchez JC: Childhood obesity in the year 2001. *Endocrinologist* 5:296–306, 2001
6. Friedland O, Nemet D, Gorodnitsky N, Wolach B, Eliakim A: Obesity and lipid profiles in children and adolescents. *J Pediatr Endocrinol Metab* 15:1011–1016, 2002
7. Epstein LH, Myers MD, Raynor HA, Saelens BE: Treatment of pediatric obesity. *Pediatrics* 101:554–570, 1998
8. Jeffrey RW: Community programs for obesity prevention: the Minnesota Heart Health Program. *Obesity Res* 3 (Suppl. 2):283S–288S, 1995

9. Gortmaker SL, Peterson K, Wiecha J, Sobol AM, Dixit S, Fox MK, et al.: Reducing obesity via a school-based interdisciplinary intervention among youth: Planet Health. *Arch Pediatr Adolesc Med* 153:409–418, 1999

10. Hoelscher DM, Kelder SH, Murray N, Cribb PW, Conroy J, Parcel GS: Dissemination and adoption of the Child and Adolescents Trial for Cardiovascular Health (CATCH): a case study in Texas. *J Public Health Manag Pract* 7:90–100, 2001

11. Trevino RP, Pugh JA, Hernandez AE, Menchaca VD, Ramirez RR, Mendoza M: Bienestar: a diabetes risk-factor prevention program. *J Sch Health* 68:62–67, 1998

12. Cook VV, Hurley JS: Prevention of type 2 diabetes in childhood. *Clin Pediatr* 37:123–129, 1998

13. Gortmaker SL, Cheung LWY, Peterson KE, Chomitz G, Cradle JH, Dart H, et al.: Impact of a school-based interdisciplinary intervention on diet and physical activity among urban primary school children. *Arch Pediatr Adolesc Med* 153:975–983, 1999

14. Macaulay AC, Paradis G, Potvin L, Cross EJ, Saad-Haddad C, McComber A, et al.: The Kahnawake Schools Diabetes Prevention Project: intervention, evaluation and baseline results of a diabetes primary prevention program with a native community in Canada. *Prev Med* 26:779–790, 1997

15. Robinson TN: Reducing children's television viewing to prevent obesity: a randomized controlled trial. *JAMA* 282:1561–1567, 1999

16. Teufel NI, Ritenbaugh CK: Development of a primary prevention program: insight gained in the Zuni Diabetes Prevention Program. *Clin Pediatr (Phila)* 37:131–141, 1998

17. von Kries R, Koletzko B, Sauerwald T, von Mutius E, Barnert D, Grunert V, et al.: Breast feeding and obesity: cross sectional study. *BMJ* 319:147–150, 1999

18. Freedman DS, Khan LK, Dietz WH, Srinivasan SR, Berenson GS: Relationship of childhood obesity to coronary heart disease risk factors in adulthood: the Bogalusa Heart Study. *Pediatrics* 108:712–718, 2001

19. Pan XR, Li GW, Hu YH, Wang JX, Yang WY, An ZX, et al.: Effects of diet and exercise in preventing NIDDM in people with impaired glucose tolerance: the Da Qing IGT and Diabetes Study. *Diabetes Care* 20:537–544, 1997

20. Tuomilehto J, Lindstrom J, Eriksson JG, Valle TT, Hamalainen H, Ilanne-Parikka P, et al.: Prevention of type 2 diabetes mellitus by changes in lifestyle among subjects with impaired glucose tolerance. *N Engl J Med* 344:1343–1350, 2001

21. Swinburn BA, Metcalf PA, Ley SJ: Long-term (5-year) effects of a reduced-fat diet intervention in individuals with glucose intolerance. *Diabetes Care* 24:619–624, 2001

22. Diabetes Prevention Program Research Group: Reduction in the incidence of type 2 diabetes with lifestyle intervention or metformin. *N Engl J Med* 346:393–403, 2002

23. Epstein LH, Valoski AM, Kalarchian MA, McCurley J: Do children lose and maintain weight easier than adults: a comparison of child and parent weight changes from six months to ten years. *Obes Res* 3:411–417, 1995

24. Levine MD, Ringham RM, Kalarchian MA, Wisniewski L, Marcus MD: Is family-based behavioral weight control appropriate for severe pediatric obesity? *Int J Eat Disord* 30:318–328, 2001

25. Daniels S: Pharmacological treatment of obesity in paediatric patients. *Paediatr Drugs* 3:405–410, 2001

26. Freemark M, Bursey D: The effects of metformin on body mass index and glucose tolerance in obese adolescents with fasting hyperinsulinemia and a family history of type 2 diabetes. *Pediatrics* 107:E55, 2001

27. Segal DG, Sanchez JC: Childhood obesity in the year 2001. *Endocrinologist* 11:296–306, 2001

28. Strauss RS, Bradley LJ, Brolin RE: Gastric bypass surgery in adolescents with morbid obesity. *J Pediatr* 138:499–504, 2001

CHAPTER 7

Treatment

INTRODUCTION

The emergence of type 2 diabetes in children and adolescents has required that specialists familiar with the management of type 1 diabetes in children recognize the vast differences between the treatment challenges of these two disorders (1).

- **Socioeconomic.** Type 1 diabetes is distributed throughout the population proportionate to socioeconomic distribution, whereas type 2 diabetes disproportionately affects individuals with fewer resources, e.g., single parents, less educated parents, and individuals who are less well insured (2).
- **Age.** Type 1 diabetes occurs throughout childhood, when parental influence is predominant, whereas type 2 diabetes occurs typically in adolescence, when peer influence predominates.
- **Family experience.** Only ~5% of families with a child with type 1 diabetes have family experience with the disease, whereas ≥90% of families of the child with type 2 diabetes have such experience. The typical failure of these family members to control weight and glycemia, with resultant complications, can lead to despair and resignation.
- **Treatment priorities.** In type 1 diabetes, major lifestyle modification, beyond insulin administration and glucose monitoring, is only needed in individuals who are overweight and inactive. For all patients with type 2 diabetes, the emphasis is primarily on lifestyle modification.
- **Effects of technology.** Technological advancements have revolutionized the management of type 1 diabetes (e.g., insulin purity and delivery systems, blood glucose monitoring, insulin analogs) and have led

to the imminence of an artificial pancreas and the likelihood of islet cell replacement. In contrast, technological advances in entertainment, labor-saving devices, and transportation, together with an economic environment that makes calorically dense food increasingly available, desirable, and inexpensive, have led to the emergence of type 2 diabetes in children.

TREATMENT GOALS

■ Overall goals (3)
   ● normalize glycemia and A1C
   ● decrease weight
   ● increase exercise capability
   ● control hypertension and hyperlipidemia
   ● reduce/resolve acanthosis nigricans
■ Importance of treatment
   ● Because of the multitude of cardiovascular risk factors associated with insulin resistance, type 2 diabetes is likely to be associated with earlier severe complications than type 1 diabetes diagnosed in childhood (4,5).
   ● The insidious onset in much of type 2 diabetes, and the unknown duration of pre-diabetes preceding diagnosis, may, as in adults, be associated with vascular disease already present at diagnosis. This is suggested by experience with 100 Pima children and adolescents with type 2 diabetes (6).
      □ At diagnosis
         ○ 7% had high cholesterol (≥200 mg/dl)
         ○ 18% had hypertension (BP ≥140/90 mmHg)
         ○ 22% had microalbuminuria (alb/Cr ≥30)
      □ After 10 years
         ○ mean A1C was 12%
         ○ 60% had microalbuminuria
         ○ 17% had macroalbuminuria (alb/Cr ≥300)
   ● Reducing complications may require more stringent control in insulin-resistant patients with type 2 diabetes than in patients with type 1 diabetes, with especially diligent attention to comorbidities, as suggested by the United Kingdom Prospective Diabetes Study (7,8), which demonstrated
      □ 25% decrease in the risk for microvascular complications associated with a reduction of average A1C from 7.9 to 7.0%
      □ 37% decrease in the risk of macrovascular disease with BP <144/82 mmHg (stroke decreased 44%, heart failure decreased 36%)

TREATMENT PRINCIPLES

- Diet and exercise form the foundation of treatment, with normal glycemia the primary measurable goal.
- Weight loss is the most effective treatment for insulin resistance, the basic cause of type 2 diabetes.
- Adolescents have more problems with adherence to treatment programs than other age-groups because of
  - the struggle for independence and autonomy
  - a desire to be like their peers, i.e., eat what they eat, engage in passive endeavors, and not take medication branding them as different
  - risk-taking behaviors for excitement and because they feel invulnerable
  - high rate of depression
- Adherence must be assessed at each clinic visit using
  - a structured, detailed interview of daily routine, including medication intake, blood glucose monitoring, food habits, and exercise
  - a refill history from pharmacy, if on medication
- Attaining treatment goals requires behavioral modification and involvement of the family, with a team approach. In addition to the physician and diabetes nurse educator, the team should include a psychologist or other trained counselor (e.g., a social worker), a dietitian, and an exercise specialist.

BEHAVIORAL CHANGE

- Principles of behavioral change are discussed in Chapter 6. The treatment team requires inclusion of a psychologist or social worker for long-term success.
- Children frequently consume nondiet soft drinks and juices in large quantities. Substitute water or diet soft drinks and use sugar substitutes for sweetening tea or Kool-Aid.
- Develop and encourage an achievable daily exercise program.
- Break the vicious cycle of increased weight–increased torpor–decreased activity–increased weight. The most effective method is turning off the television.
- A relatively small reduction in weight, especially if accomplished by increased activity, can restore euglycemia and decrease hyperinsulinemia.
- Table 13 outlines the stages of change involved in behavioral modification.

TABLE 13. Stages of Change Involved in Behavioral Modification

Concept	Definition	Application
Pre-contemplation	Unaware of problem; has no intention of changing in the near future (next 6 months) and may deny need for change. "Everyone in our family is big."	Increase awareness of need for change, personalize information on risks or benefits
Contemplation	Thinking about change in the near future; knows there is an issue but is not ready to change; there may be intent to change in the next 6 months. "I've heard that some overweight kids are getting diabetes. But I don't think I can handle going on a diet."	Motivate, encourage to make specific plans
Preparation	Making a plan to change; knows what he or she wants to do; is seeking more information, planning, even starting to change; may tell family and friends; there is an intent to change in the near future. "I found out that if I lose some weight, this smudge on my neck will fade. I've talked to my mom about it. . . ."	Assist in developing concrete action plans, setting gradual goals
Action	Implementation of specific action plans; making changes in the environment to support the change. Relapse is normal. This stage may last as long as 6 months. "I'm walking three times a week for half an hour. I've quit drinking sodas. . . ."	Assist with feedback, problem solving, social support, reinforcement
Maintenance	Continuation of desirable actions; or repeating periodic recommended step(s); may last 6 months to 5 years; some add a sixth stage, termination; "I lost 10 pounds. The smudge on my neck went away. I am going to keep on walking and eating better."	Assist in coping, reminders, finding alternatives, avoiding relapses (as apply)

This outline comes from a comprehensive and informative handbook prepared by the University of Texas Health Science Center at San Antonio/Department of Pediatrics and The Children's Center at the Texas Diabetes Institute. The handbook is titled *Kids, Teens, and Type 2 Diabetes: What You Need to Know: An Essential Reference for School Nurses.* (Contact 210-358-7550 or 210-567-7481, e-mail: livingstonj@uthscsa.edu, for more information.)

AVAILABLE HYPOGLYCEMIC AGENTS

- Diet and exercise modification remains effective in controlling blood glucose longer than a few months in <15% of patients. If and when this intervention fails, treatment with hypoglycemic agents is indicated. There are no U.S. Food and Drug Administration–approved specific indications for the use of oral hypoglycemic agents other than metformin in children.
- The aim of pharmacological therapy is to decrease insulin resistance, increase insulin secretion, or slow postprandial glucose absorption. Table 14 examines the effects of each of the hypoglycemic agents discussed in this section.

TABLE 14. Available Hypoglycemic Agents

Drug Type	Action	Effect on Blood Glucose	Risk of Low Blood Glucose	Weight Increase	Lipid Decrease
Biguanides (metformin)	↓ hepatic glucose output ↑ hepatic insulin sensitivity	++	0	0	+
Sulfonylureas	↑ insulin secretion and sensitivity	++	++	++	0
Meglitinide (repaglinide)	Creates short term ↑ in insulin secretion	++	+	+	0
α-Glucosidase inhibitors (acarbose, miglitol)	Slows hydrolysis and absorption of complex CHO	+	0	0	+
Thiazolidinediones (rosiglitazone, pioglitazone)	↑ insulin sensitivity in muscle and fat tissue	++	0	+	+
Insulin	↓ hepatic glucose output; overcomes insulin resistance	+++	++	++	+

Biguanides (9)

- Action is on insulin receptors in liver, muscle, and fat tissue.
- Hepatic glucose production is reduced by decreasing gluconeogenesis.
- Insulin-stimulated glucose uptake is increased in muscle and fat.
- Anorexic effect can promote weight loss.
- Long-term use is associated with a 1–2% reduction in A1C.
- High rate of side effects limits compliance in adolescents:
  - abdominal pain, nausea, vomiting, diarrhea, bloating, and nonpalatability
  - especially problematic if breakfast skipped, a common practice in adolescence, and metformin taken on an empty stomach
  - fewer gastrointestinal side effects with long-acting preparation
- An in-depth history of medication intake, including refill history from the pharmacy, may explain the lack of therapeutic effect.
- Biguanides must not be given to patients with renal impairment, hepatic disease, or cardiac or respiratory insufficiency or who are receiving radiographic contrast materials because of risk of lactic acidosis. Alcohol ingestion also increases the risk of lactic acidosis.
- Metformin is the only hypoglycemic agent approved for use in pediatric patients, based on a multicenter trial (10):
  - 82 previously untreated 8- to 16-year-old patients randomized to metformin or placebo
  - initial dose of 500 mg twice daily with breakfast and dinner, increased to 2,000 mg/day over 2 weeks
  - few placebo cases remained by 16 weeks of study because of the need to treat elevated blood glucose and A1C
  - after ≥4 months
    - mean fasting glucose change from baseline −44 mg/dl metformin, +20 mg/dl placebo
    - adjusted mean A1C: 7.5% metformin, 8.6% placebo
  - no weight gain, with a modest decrease in weight in some patients, and improved lipid profiles
  - no serious adverse events
- Metformin may normalize ovulatory abnormalities in girls with PCOS and increase pregnancy risk.

Sulfonylurea and Meglitinide/Repaglinide (11)

- Action is to increase insulin secretion, and they are, thus, most useful when there is residual β-cell function.

■ Sulfonylureas bind to receptors on the K$^+$/ATP channel complex. (With rising plasma glucose concentration, there is rapid phosphorylation of glucose to glucose-6-phosphate, which is rapidly metabolized to convert ADP to ATP. When the ATP-to-ADP ratio increases, K$^+$ channels close, resulting in depolarization of the adjacent cell membrane, opening Ca^{2+} channels. The greater the plasma glucose concentration, the more K$^+$ channels that close and Ca^{2+} channels that open, increasing insulin release.)

■ Meglitinide and repaglinide bind to separate sites on the K$^+$/ATP channel complex.

■ Activation of ATP, or binding by sulfonylurea or meglitinide, causes K$^+$ channels to close.

■ ATP binding sites equilibrate rapidly, whereas sulfonylurea sites equilibrate slowly and binding persists for prolonged periods; thus, traditional sulfonylureas have prolonged effects.

■ Meglitinide has an intermediate equilibration and binding duration and is thus used for rapid enhancement of insulin secretion, e.g., before meals.

■ Major adverse effects of sulfonylureas are hypoglycemia, which can be prolonged, and weight gain. Meglitinide is associated with less and briefer hypoglycemia.

Thiazolidinediones (Glitazones) (12)

■ Action is to increase insulin sensitivity in muscle, adipose, and liver tissue.

■ Glitazones bind to nuclear proteins, activating the peroxisome proliferator activator receptor (PPAR)-γ, an orphan steroid receptor particularly abundant in adipocytes, ultimately increasing formation of proteins involved in the nuclear-based actions of insulin, including cell growth, adipose cell differentiation, regulation of insulin receptor activity, and glucose transport into the cell.

■ Long-term treatment is associated with a reduction in A1C of 0.5–1.3%.

■ Side effects include edema, weight gain, and anemia.

■ Liver enzymes were elevated in ~1% of patients taking the original member of this group, troglitazone, with fatalities resulting in its withdrawal.

■ Newer glitazones, rosiglitazone and pioglitazone, appear not to have significant hepatotoxicity.

■ Binding of the glitazones to PPAR-γ is ubiquitous, including arterial walls with muscle, affecting muscle cell growth and migration in response to growth factors (13).

- Glitazones also improve lipid profiles (decreased LDL cholesterol and triglyceride and increased HDL cholesterol). This effect and that on muscle could be important in reducing macrovascular disease associated with type 2 diabetes.
- No published data are available on the use of rosiglitazone or pioglitazone in pediatric patients with type 2 diabetes. Pediatric trials are underway.

α-Glucosidase Inhibitors (14)

- α-Glucosidase inhibitors (acarbose, miglitol) reduce the absorption of carbohydrates in the upper small intestine by inhibiting the breakdown of oligosaccharides, thereby delaying absorption in the lower small intestine.
- The postprandial rise of plasma glucose is reduced.
- Long-term therapy is associated with a 0.5–1.0% reduction in A1C.
- The frequent side effect of flatulence makes these agents unacceptable for most children and adolescents.
- Pediatric trials are underway.

Insulin

- Studies in adults indicate that ~50% of β-cell function is already lost by the time of diagnosis and that most individuals require insulin 6–7 years later.
- In one study of 49 African American and Caribbean Hispanic children with type 2 diabetes, 50% were able to maintain good glycemic control without insulin 5 years after diagnosis (15).
- Despite hyperinsulinemia and insulin resistance, relatively small doses of supplemental insulin are often effective.
- The only side effects of insulin are hypoglycemia, which has not been common in patients with type 2 diabetes treated with insulin, and weight gain, a substantial problem in this population.
- Insulin glargine, a long-acting insulin analog without peak effects, may be useful in patients with type 2 diabetes, in combination with premeal meglitinide, and in patients who are unwilling to take metformin (16,17).

TREATMENT RECOMMENDATIONS

Treatment is determined by symptoms, severity of hyperglycemia, and presence or absence of ketosis/ketoacidosis (Fig. 10).

- As in type 1 diabetes, individuals with symptoms, particularly vomiting, can deteriorate rapidly.

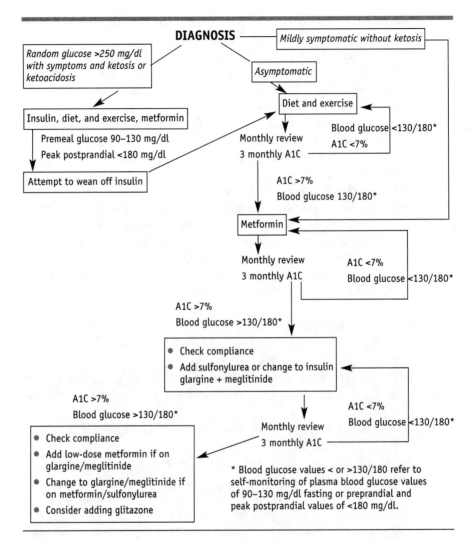

FIGURE 10. Therapy decision tree for type 2 diabetes in children and adolescents. The A1C and glucose goals shown are those recommended by the ADA for adults with diabetes (18). The recommendations state that goals should be individualized, that certain populations, including children, require special considerations, and that postprandial glucose may be targeted if A1C goals are not met despite reaching preprandial glucose goals.

- Ketoacidosis is treated the same as in type 1 diabetes, even if there is no question that one is dealing with type 2 disease.
- An oral agent (e.g., metformin or premeal meglitinide) should be started when ketoacidosis is resolved, and insulin should be continued, using starting doses of 0.5 units/kg/day insulin given as 60–70% in the morning and 30–40% in the evening.
- Initial distribution of insulin is similar to that given to patients with type 1 diabetes and adjusted based on blood glucose values obtained before and 2 hours after meals and at bedtime until blood glucose levels are in the target range.
- When target plasma blood glucose goals of 90–130 mg/dl premeal and <180 between meals are attained, insulin can be reduced and stopped over a period of days while monitoring blood glucose levels.
- Metformin should be the first oral agent used. It has the advantage over sulfonylureas of similar reduction in A1C without the risk of hypoglycemia. Furthermore, weight is either decreased or remains stable, and LDL cholesterol and triglyceride levels decrease.
- Failure to achieve glycemic and A1C goals with metformin over 3–6 months indicates the need to add a sulfonylurea or insulin.
- Insulin glargine is used by some pediatric diabetologists for type 2 diabetes, in combination with premeal meglitinide.
  - Glargine has a long duration of action, up to 24 hours, with little or no peak effect, thus acting as a basal insulin to inhibit hepatic glucose production.
  - The short-acting meglitinide results in acute insulin release, providing coverage for meals.
  - This regimen permits flexibility in the timing of meals, which is important to adolescents.
  - Hypoglycemic risk is lower than with previous forms of intermediate-acting insulin, and patient preference in adults is high (17).
- Glitazones may be used in older adolescents. However, there are no studies available in young patients.
- Type 2 diabetes is a result of both insulin resistance and failure of compensatory insulin production by the β-cells.
  - Thus, use of multiple complementary agents to target both problems is warranted when monotherapy with metformin fails.
  - Glitazones and metformin improve insulin sensitivity, whereas sulfonylureas and meglitinide stimulate insulin secretion.
  - Pills combining sulfonylurea and metformin are available. These pills can enhance compliance.

- Over the course of 6–10 years, almost all adults with type 2 diabetes will require insulin. No data are available for pediatric patients.
- Insulin is most effective when used in combination with an agent that increases insulin sensitivity (metformin, glitazones) or as the combination described above (insulin glargine, meglitinide). Because of the insulin resistance in type 2 diabetes, hypoglycemia is not as prevalent as in insulin-treated type 1 diabetes.
- No oral agent should be used during pregnancy, highlighting the importance of counseling adolescents with type 2 diabetes about sexuality and pregnancy.
- Self-monitoring of blood glucose (SMBG) should be performed routinely and during periods of acute illness or when symptoms of hyperglycemia or hypoglycemia occur. Patients on insulin or sulfonylureas also need to monitor for asymptomatic hypoglycemia. Although optimal frequency of SMBG is four times daily, frequency must be individualized and include a combination of fasting/preprandial and postprandial glucose measurements (19).
- A1C concentration should be assayed quarterly. If metabolic control is unsatisfactory, referral to a dietitian with knowledge and experience in nutritional management of children with diabetes and to a psychologist/social worker who has experience in behavior modification techniques for this population is indicated.
- Changes in treatment regimen should only be made after dealing with compliance and behavioral issues and should be based on reliable blood glucose testing.
- Dietary recommendations should be culturally appropriate, sensitive to family resources, and provided to all caregivers.

TREATMENT OF COMORBIDITIES

Hypertension

- Hypertension is an independent risk factor for the development of albuminuria, retinopathy, and cardiovascular disease in type 2 diabetes.
- BP is an important factor in the early appearance of atherosclerotic lesions in children and adolescents (20).
  - The Bogalusa Heart Study of autopsy findings in children 2–15 years of age (21) described
    - fatty streaks in coronary arteries in 50%
    - raised fibrous plaques in coronary arteries in 8%

      ☐ lesions correlating with BMI, systolic and diastolic BP, and lipid
abnormalities (elevated total and LDL-cholesterol and triglycerides)
- The Pathological Determinants of Atherosclerosis in Youth Study of
>3,000 autopsies of males and females 15–34 years old dying of ex-
ternal causes (22) described
      ☐ lesions in all aortas and half of right coronary arteries
      ☐ lesions in 7% of aortas and 12% of right coronary arteries in the
age-group 15–19 years
      ☐ every 1 SD increase of VLDL and LDL-cholesterol associated with
surface involvement increase of 5%
      ☐ increased BP associated with doubling of the prevalence of raised le-
sions involving >5% of the intimal surface
■ Carotid artery intima thickening, a marker of generalized atherosclerosis
and a predictor of future cardiovascular events in adults, was increased
in 50 children with type 1 diabetes compared with 35 age-, sex-, and
BMI-matched control subjects (23).
- Mean age was 11 ± 2 years and duration of diabetes 4.4 ± 3 years.
- Systolic BP and high LDL cholesterol were significantly associated
with the degree of carotid intima-media thickness.
- There was no effect of age, sex, BMI, or A1C.
■ Studies in adults have shown a decreased incidence of major cardiovascular events with antihypertensive therapy.
- Heart Outcomes Prevention Evaluation Study (24)
      ☐ included 9,297 patients >55 years old at high risk for cardiovascular
disease, including 3,577 with type 2 diabetes and no previous history
of ischemic heart disease
      ☐ observed a 22% reduction in cardiovascular endpoints and a signif-
icantly decreased risk of microvascular complications (6.4 vs. 7.6%)
with the use of an ACE inhibitor compared with placebo, despite
only a 3-mmHg decrease in systolic BP and a 2-mmHg decrease in
diastolic BP
      ☐ suggested that ACE inhibitors have beneficial effects independent of
the effects on BP
- Hypertension Optimal Treatment Trial (25)
      ☐ randomly assigned 18,790 patients age 50–80 years with diastolic
BP between 100 and 115 mmHg to target BP of ≤80 mmHg
($n = 6,262$), ≤85 mmHg ($n = 6,264$), or ≤90 mmHg ($n = 6,264$)
      ☐ found decrease of major cardiovascular events by >50% with target
diastolic BP ≤80 mmHg compared with ≤90 mmHg in the 1,501 patients who had diabetes at study onset

- In the United Kingdom Prospective Diabetes Study, hypertension control was more important than blood glucose control in decreasing the frequency of cardiac events (8).
- A study of 589 children with type 1 diabetes onset before 17 years of age has shown increased risk of nephropathy, proliferative retinopathy, peripheral neuropathy, cardiovascular disease, and peripheral arterial disease with high BP over the 10 years after diagnosis (26).
  - Systolic BP ≥120–129 mmHg conferred a relative risk of cardiovascular disease of 2.5.
  - Systolic BP ≥130 mmHg conferred a relative risk for nephropathy of 2.3, for peripheral neuropathy 4.0, and for proliferative retinopathy 2.7.
  - Diastolic BP ≥85 mmHg conferred a relative risk for nephropathy of 2.5, for peripheral neuropathy 2.0, and for proliferative retinopathy 2.4.
  - The relative risk of proliferative retinopathy increased to 4.6 if diastolic BP was ≥90 mmHg.
- BP should be measured at each quarterly examination.
  - BP should be taken with the patient resting in the sitting position. The first and fifth Korotkoff sounds should be recorded as systolic and diastolic BP.
  - BP should be taken at least twice to minimize the "white coat effect" of the stress of the medical setting.
  - Elevations should be rechecked at least twice at weekly intervals.
- Body size is the most important determinant of BP in children and adolescents. Therefore, the 90th and 95th percentiles for BP for each age are given in relation to height percentiles in Tables 15 and 16 (27).
- Persistent BP >90th percentile for age, sex, and height should initially be treated with diet and exercise.
- If BP remains elevated after 3 months of diet and exercise prescription, organic causes of hypertension need to be ruled out and the use of an ACE inhibitor considered.
- ACE inhibitors
  - block ACE, decreasing the production of angiotensin II, a potent vasoconstrictor
  - block the breakdown of bradykinin by ACE, increasing the levels of bradykinin, a potent vasodilator
  - enhance the vasodilator effect of nitrous oxide via bradykinin
  - inhibit platelet aggregation and endothelin production, a procoagulant fibrinolysis inhibitor

TABLE 15. Levels for the 90th and 95th Percentiles of BP for Girls Age 1–17 Years by Percentiles of Height

Age	Height Percentiles* → BP† ↓	Systolic BP (mmHg)							Diastolic BP (mmHg)						
		5%	10%	25%	50%	75%	90%	95%	5%	10%	25%	50%	75%	90%	95%
1	90th	97	98	99	100	102	103	104	53	53	53	54	55	56	56
	95th	101	102	103	104	105	107	107	57	57	57	58	59	60	60
2	90th	99	99	100	102	103	104	105	57	57	58	58	59	60	61
	95th	102	103	104	105	107	108	109	61	61	62	62	63	64	65
3	90th	100	100	102	103	104	105	106	61	61	61	62	63	63	64
	95th	104	104	105	107	108	109	110	65	65	65	66	67	67	68
4	90th	101	102	103	104	106	107	108	63	63	64	65	65	66	67
	95th	105	106	107	108	109	111	111	67	67	68	69	69	70	71
5	90th	103	103	104	106	107	108	109	65	66	66	67	68	68	69
	95th	107	107	108	110	111	112	113	69	70	70	71	72	72	73
6	90th	104	105	106	107	109	110	111	67	67	68	69	69	70	71
	95th	108	109	110	111	112	114	114	71	71	72	73	73	74	75
7	90th	106	107	108	109	110	112	112	69	69	69	70	71	72	72
	95th	110	110	112	113	114	115	116	73	73	73	74	75	76	76
8	90th	108	109	110	111	112	113	114	70	70	71	71	72	73	74
	95th	112	112	113	115	116	117	118	74	74	75	75	76	77	78

Age	BP Percentile	Systolic BP by Height Percentile							Diastolic BP by Height Percentile						
9	90th	110	110	112	113	114	115	116	71	72	72	73	74	74	75
	95th	114	114	115	117	118	119	120	75	76	76	77	78	78	79
10	90th	112	112	114	115	116	117	118	73	73	73	74	75	76	76
	95th	116	116	117	119	120	121	122	77	77	77	78	79	80	80
11	90th	114	114	116	117	118	119	120	74	74	75	75	76	77	77
	95th	118	118	119	121	122	123	124	78	78	79	79	80	81	81
12	90th	116	116	118	119	120	121	122	75	75	76	76	77	78	78
	95th	120	120	121	123	124	125	126	79	79	80	80	81	82	82
13	90th	118	118	119	121	122	123	124	76	76	77	78	78	79	80
	95th	121	122	123	125	126	127	128	80	80	81	82	82	83	84
14	90th	119	120	121	122	124	125	126	77	77	78	79	79	80	81
	95th	123	124	125	126	128	129	130	81	81	82	83	83	84	85
15	90th	121	121	122	124	125	126	127	78	78	79	79	80	81	82
	95th	124	125	126	128	129	130	131	82	82	83	83	84	85	86
16	90th	122	122	123	125	126	127	128	79	79	79	80	81	82	82
	95th	125	126	127	128	130	131	132	83	83	83	84	85	86	86
17	90th	122	123	124	125	126	128	128	79	79	79	80	81	82	82
	95th	126	126	127	129	130	131	132	83	83	83	84	85	86	86

* Height percentile determined by standard growth curves.
† BP percentile determined by a single measurement

TABLE 16. Levels for the 90th and 95th Percentiles of BP for Boys Age 1–17 Years by Percentiles of Height

Age	BP†	Systolic BP (mmHg)							Diastolic BP (mmHg)						
Height Percentiles* →		5%	10%	25%	50%	75%	90%	95%	5%	10%	25%	50%	75%	90%	95%
1	90th	94	95	97	98	100	102	102	50	51	52	53	54	54	55
	95th	98	99	101	102	104	106	106	55	55	56	57	58	59	59
2	90th	98	99	100	102	104	105	106	55	55	56	57	58	59	59
	95th	101	102	104	106	108	109	110	59	59	60	61	62	63	63
3	90th	100	101	103	105	107	108	109	59	59	60	61	62	63	63
	95th	104	105	107	109	111	112	113	63	63	64	65	66	67	67
4	90th	102	103	105	107	109	110	111	62	62	63	64	65	66	66
	95th	106	107	109	111	113	114	115	66	67	67	68	69	70	71
5	90th	104	105	106	108	110	112	112	65	65	66	67	68	69	69
	95th	108	109	110	112	114	115	116	69	70	70	71	72	73	74
6	90th	105	106	108	110	111	113	114	67	68	69	70	70	71	72
	95th	109	110	112	114	115	117	117	72	72	73	74	75	76	76
7	90th	106	107	109	111	113	114	115	69	70	71	72	72	73	74
	95th	110	111	113	115	116	118	119	74	74	75	76	77	78	78
8	90th	107	108	110	112	114	115	116	71	71	72	73	74	75	75
	95th	111	112	114	116	118	119	120	75	76	76	77	78	79	80

Age	Percentile	Systolic BP							Diastolic BP						
9	90th	109	110	112	113	115	117	117	72	73	73	74	75	76	77
	95th	113	114	116	117	119	121	121	76	77	78	79	80	80	81
10	90th	110	112	113	115	117	118	119	73	74	74	75	76	77	78
	95th	114	115	117	119	121	122	123	77	78	79	80	80	81	82
11	90th	112	113	115	117	119	120	121	74	74	75	76	77	78	78
	95th	116	117	119	121	123	124	125	78	79	79	80	81	82	83
12	90th	115	116	117	119	121	123	123	75	75	76	77	78	78	79
	95th	119	120	121	123	125	126	127	79	79	80	81	82	83	83
13	90th	117	118	120	122	124	125	126	75	76	76	77	78	79	80
	95th	121	122	124	126	128	129	130	79	80	81	82	83	83	84
14	90th	120	121	123	125	126	128	128	76	76	77	78	79	80	80
	95th	124	125	127	128	130	132	132	80	81	81	82	83	84	85
15	90th	123	124	125	127	129	131	131	77	77	78	79	80	81	81
	95th	127	128	129	131	133	134	135	81	82	83	83	84	85	86
16	90th	125	126	128	130	132	133	134	79	79	80	81	82	82	83
	95th	129	130	132	134	136	137	138	83	83	84	85	86	87	87
17	90th	128	129	131	133	134	136	136	81	81	82	83	84	85	85
	95th	132	133	135	136	138	140	140	85	85	86	87	88	89	89

* Height percentile determined by standard growth curves.

† BP percentile determined by a single measurement

- inhibit smooth muscle proliferation, with decreased plaque rupture and subsequent thrombosis
- slow progression of retinopathy and nephropathy
- The ADA recommends treating to maintain a BP of <130/80 mmHg (28). Because albuminuria confers additional cardiovascular and microvascular risk, goals of therapy are a BP of <120/75 mmHg if the albumin excretion rate is >30 mg/day or >30 mg/g creatinine (29).
- Some practitioners use ACE inhibitors prophylactically, as in type 1 diabetes, because of the high risk for hypertension in type 2 diabetes.

Hyperlipidemia

Reduction of hyperlipidemia decreases the risk of coronary events in patients with diabetes. Coronary events are the major cause of premature mortality in type 2 diabetes.

- Studies in adults
  - The Scandinavian Simvastatin Survival Study of 4,242 adult subjects, 202 of whom had diabetes, demonstrated that HMG-CoA inhibitors (statins) decreased LDL cholesterol 36%, with a 55% risk reduction in major coronary events and a 43% reduction in mortality in the diabetes cohort (30).
  - The Cholesterol and Recurrent Events (CARE) Trial of 4,159 adult subjects, 586 of whom had diabetes, found that pravastatin decreased LDL cholesterol by 27%, with a 22% reduction in coronary heart disease risk in the diabetes cohort (31).
  - In the Medical Research Council (U.K.) Heart Protection Study (32)
    - □ 20,536 adults with increased risk of coronary heart disease were followed for 5 years
    - □ an ~25% risk reduction of cardiovascular events was seen for each level of LDL cholesterol reduction (<100, ≥100, <130, and ≥130 mg/dl) with simvastatin compared with placebo, even when the initial LDL cholesterol concentration was normal (<110 mg/dl)
- Study in children: The Pittsburgh Epidemiology of Diabetes Complications Study (26)
  - 10-year study of individuals with type 1 diabetes onset before or during adolescence
  - strong relationship found between lipid levels and risk of microvascular and cardiovascular disease
  - relative risk of cardiovascular disease 1.8 with LDL cholesterol >100 mg/dl and 2.3 with level >130 mg/dl

- relative risks for cardiovascular disease 2.5 with triglyceride >90 mg/dl and 3.3 with level >150 mg/dl
- Treatment
  - Lipid levels and urine albumin excretion should be checked at diagnosis and annually or more often if elevated, and the effect of intervention needs to be monitored.
  - The ADA recommends that adults begin treatment with diet and exercise when LDL cholesterol is ≥100 mg/dl and triglycerides are ≥150 mg/dl (33).
  - Guidelines for children are to treat LDL cholesterol >130 mg/dl, with a target of 110 mg/dl (34). However, evidence that atherosclerosis begins in childhood and that statin treatment lowers cardiovascular risk in adults supports a more aggressive approach, i.e., that adult guidelines be followed, particularly in adolescents with type 2 diabetes.
  - Hyperlipidemia may improve with exercise, weight loss, and glycemic control.
  - A reduced-fat diet consistent with step 1 American Heart Association guidelines is appropriate.
  - Isolated elevations of triglycerides should be treated with fibric acid derivatives, such as gemfibrozil.
  - Failure to normalize lipids after 2–3 months of dietary and diabetes control efforts requires addition of lipid-lowering medications.
  - Bile acid binding resins are the only drugs currently approved for treatment of dyslipidemia in children; they are unpalatable with very poor adherence.
  - Niacin is associated with flushing, also resulting in poor compliance.
  - The most commonly used lipid-lowering agents in pediatric patients, however, are the HMG-CoA reductase inhibitors (statins).
    - Studies have not shown an increase in liver or CPK abnormalities with these agents compared with placebo.
    - Thus far, experience with children and adolescents over a 10-year period in the University of Florida Lipid Clinic for Children indicates effectiveness and safety.
    - These agents are contraindicated in pregnancy or with the risk of pregnancy.

Other Considerations (19)

- A dilated eye examination should be performed annually.
- Monitoring lipids, urinary albumin excretion, and eyes, in contrast to recommendations for type 1 diabetes in children, should begin at diagnosis.

REFERENCES

1. Rosenbloom AL: Increasing incidence of type 2 diabetes mellitus in children and adolescents: treatment considerations. *Pediatr Drugs* 4:209–221, 2002
2. Pinhas-Hamiel O, Standiford D, Hamiel D, Dolan LM, Cohen R, Zeitler PS: The type 2 family: a setting for development and treatment of adolescent type 2 diabetes mellitus. *Arch Pediatr Adolesc Med* 153:1063–1067, 1999
3. Silverstein JH, Rosenbloom AL: Treatment of type 2 diabetes in children and adolescents. *J Ped Endocrinol Metab* 13:1403–1409, 2000
4. Yokoyama H, Okudaira M, Otani T, Watanabe C, Takaike H, Miuira J, et al.: High incidence of diabetic nephropathy in early-onset Japanese NIDDM patients: risk analysis. *Diabetes Care* 21:1080–1085, 1998
5. Hu FB, Stampfer MJ, Haffner SM, Solomon CG, Willett WC, Manson JE: Elevated risk of cardiovascular disease prior to clinical diagnosis of type 2 diabetes. *Diabetes Care* 25:1129–1134, 2002
6. Fagot-Campagna A, Knowler WC, Pettitt DJ: Type 2 diabetes in Pima Indian Children: cardiovascular risk factors at diagnosis and 10 years later (Abstract). *Diabetes* 47 (Suppl. 1):A155, 1998
7. United Kingdom Prospective Diabetes Study Group: Intensive blood glucose control with sulphonylureas or insulin compared with conventional treatment and risk of complications in patients with type 2 diabetes (UKPDS 33). *Lancet* 352:837–853, 1998
8. United Kingdom Prospective Diabetes Study Group: Tight blood pressure control and risk of macrovascular and microvascular complications in type 2 diabetes: UKPDS 38. *BMJ* 317:703–713, 1998
9. DeFronzo RA, Goodman AM: Efficacy of metformin in patients with non-insulin dependent diabetes mellitus: the Multicenter Metformin Study Group. *N Engl J Med* 333:541–549, 1995
10. Jones K, Arslanian S, McVie R, et al.: Metformin improves glycemic control in children with type 2 diabetes. *Diabetes Care* 25:89–94, 2002
11. Lebovitz HE: Insulin secretagogues, old and new. *Diabetes Reviews* 7:139–152, 1999
12. Schwartz S, Raskin P, Fonseca V, Graveline JF: Effect of troglitazone in insulin treated patients with type 2 diabetes. *N Engl J Med* 338:861–866, 1998
13. Law RE, Goetze S, Xi XP, Jackson S, Kawano Y, Demer L, et al.: Expression and function of PPARg in rat and human vascular smooth muscle cells. *Circulation* 101:1311–1318, 2000
14. Chiasson JL, Josse RG, Hunt JA, Palmason C, Rodger NW, Ross SA, et al.: The efficacy of acarbose in the treatment of patients with non-insulin-dependent diabetes mellitus: a multicenter controlled clinical trial. *Ann Intern Med* 121:928–935, 1994
15. Grinstein G, Aponte L, Vuguin P, Saenger P, DiMartino-Nardi, J: Presentation and 5-year follow-up of noninsulin dependent diabetes mellitus (NIDDM) in

minority youth. Abstract presented at the 81st annual meeting of The Endocrine Society, San Diego, CA, June 12–15, 1999, abstract OR 25-5

16. Mudaliar S, Edelman SV: Insulin therapy in type 2 diabetes. *Endocrinol Metab Clin North Am* 30:935–982, 2001

17. Standl E: Insulin analogues-state-of-the-art. *Horm Res* 57 (Suppl. 1):40–45, 2002

18. American Diabetes Association: Standards of medical care for patients with diabetes mellitus. *Diabetes Care* 26 (Suppl. 1):S33–S50, 2003

19. American Diabetes Association: Type 2 diabetes in children and adolescents (Consensus Statement). *Diabetes Care* 23:381–389, 2000

20. National Heart, Lung, and Blood Institute: Report of the Second Task Force on Blood Pressure Control in Children: 1987. *J Pediatr* 79:1–25, 1987

21. Berenson GS, Srinivasan SR, Bao W, Newman WP, Tracy RE, Wattigney WA: Association between multiple cardiovascular risk factors and atherosclerosis in children and young adults: the Bogalusa Heart Study. *N Engl J Med* 338:1650–1656, 1998

22. Malcom GT, Oalmann MC, Strong JP: Risk factors for atherosclerosis in young subjects: the PDAY Study: Pathobiological Determinants of Atherosclerosis in Youth. *Ann N Y Acad Sci* 817:179–188, 1997

23. Jarvisalo MJ, Putto-Laurila A, Jartti L, Lehtimaki T, Solakivi T, Ronnemaa T, et al.: Carotid artery intima-media thickness in children with type 1 diabetes. *Diabetes* 51:493–498, 2002

24. Heart Outcome Prevention Evaluation (HOPE) Study Investigators: Effects of ramipril on cardiovascular and microvascular outcomes in people with diabetes mellitus. *Lancet* 255:253–259, 2000

25. Hansson L, Zanchetti A, Carruthers SG, Dahlöf B, Elmfeldt D, Julius S, Ménard J, Rahn KH, Wedel H, Westerling S, for the HOT Study Group: Effects of intensive blood-pressure lowering and low-dose aspirin in patients with hypertension: principal results of the Hypertension Optimal Treatment (HOT) randomized trial. *Lancet* 351:1755–1762, 1998

26. Orchard TJ, Forrest KYZ, Kuller LH, Becker DJ: Lipid and blood pressure treatment goals for type 1 diabetes: 10 year incidence data from the Pittsburgh Epidemiology of Complications Study. *Diabetes Care* 24:1053–1059, 2001

27. Rosner B, Prineas RJ, Loggie JM, Daniels SR: Blood pressure nomograms for children and adolescents, by height, sex, and age, in the United States. *J Pediatr* 123:871–886, 1993

28. American Diabetes Association: The treatment of hypertension in adult patients with diabetes (Technical Review). *Diabetes Care* 25:134–147, 2002

29. Joint National Committee on Prevention, Detection, Evaluation and Treatment of High Blood Pressure: The sixth report of the Joint National Committee on Prevention, Detection, Evaluation and Treatment of High Blood Pressure. *Arch Intern Med* 157:2413–2446, 1997

30. Pyorala K, Pedersen TR, Kjekshus J, Faergeman O, Olsson AG, Thorgeirsson G: Cholesterol lowering with simvastatin improves prognosis of diabetic patients with coronary artery disease. *Diabetes Care* 20:614–620, 1997

31. Goldberg RB, Mellies MJ, Sacks FM, Moye LA, Howard BV, Howard WJ, et al.: Cardiovascular events and their reduction with pravastatin in diabetic and glucose-intolerant myocardial infarction survivors with average cholesterol levels: subgroup analyses in the Cholesterol and Recurrent Events (CARE) trial: The CARE Investigators. *Circulation* 98:2513–2519, 1998

32. Heart Protection Study Collaborative Group: MRC/BHF Heart Protection Study of cholesterol lowering with simvastatin in 20,536 high risk individuals: a randomised placebo-controlled trial. *Lancet* 360:7–22, 2002

33. American Diabetes Association: Management of dyslipidemia in adults with diabetes. *Diabetes Care* 25:74–77, 2002

34. National Heart, Lung, and Blood Institute: *National Cholesterol Education Program Report of the Expert Panel on Blood Cholesterol Levels in Children and Adolescents, 1991.* Bethesda, MD, National Heart, Lung, and Blood Institute Information Center, 1991

CHAPTER 8

Patients

The patients discussed in this chapter have been selected to depict the wide range of clinical presentation and evolution of type 2 diabetes and the insulin resistance syndrome in children. No patients have been invented or had their data altered. Patient 1 has previously been described (Rosenbloom AL: Case study: an 11-year-old girl with asymptomatic diabetes. *Clinical Diabetes* 16:197–198, 1998). Patients 5 and 9 were presented at a conference at Mount Sinai School of Medicine in December 2001 by Dr. Robert R. Moghaddas and Dr. Sudha Reddy.

PATIENT 1: AN 11-YEAR-OLD PREPUBERTAL FEMALE WITH ASYMPTOMATIC DIABETES

- African-American found to have glucosuria at routine examination at a health department clinic
- random blood glucose 189 mg/dl (10.5 mmol/l)
- no health concerns, no symptoms of diabetes
- no known first-degree relatives with diabetes; disease said to run in the family by paternal grandmother
- physically inactive; only nonschool activity is participation in church
- good student in appropriate grade level
- height normal, weight 69 kg; BMI 22.6 kg/m², 90–95th percentile for age (normal for age 17.5 kg/m²)
- acanthosis nigricans in the neck folds and the axilla
- subsequent blood glucose 124 mg/dl (6.9 mmol/l) 5 hours after meal, 132 mg/dl (7.3 mmol/l) fasting; A1C 12.3%, indicative of chronic hyperglycemia

- no ketonuria
- insulin 47 μU/ml (337 pmol/l), C-peptide also elevated at 4 pg/l when glucose 181 mg/dl (10 mmol/l)
- no immunologic markers for autoimmune diabetes
- ~1-kg weight loss and no substantive change in A1C concentration (11.7%) with 3-month regimen of diet and exercise
- started on glyburide 2.5 mg/day, increasing to 5 mg/day
- A1C 10.5–13% over subsequent year
- extensive psychological and diet counseling not successful
- glyburide dose increased to 10 mg/day; despite increasing weight, A1C fell to 8% in 4 months
- deteriorating metabolic control despite introduction of troglitazone, then insulin, over the subsequent year, with A1C climbing to above 12%

Comments

- It is estimated that approximately one-third of adults with type 2 diabetes are undiagnosed. This patient's experience, a common one, suggests that there may be a substantial number of undiagnosed children as well. At 11 years of age, she had no symptoms of diabetes and no immediate family history.
- Although the patient was overweight, a member of a high-risk ethnic group, and had acanthosis nigricans (an indicator of insulin resistance), thus meeting the full criteria for testing according to ADA/American Academy of Pediatrics recommendations, were it not for the glycosuria noted on a routine examination at the health department, the diabetes might have remained undiagnosed for years.
- The A1C level of 12.3%, consistent with an average blood glucose of ~310 mg/dl (17 mmol/l), indicates longstanding disease. This is one reason why, unlike practice for children with type 1 diabetes, the indicators of microvascular complications should be assessed at diagnosis in children with type 2 diabetes. The other reason is that insulin resistance may put patients with type 2 diabetes at even greater risk for microvascular and macrovascular disease than patients with type 1 diabetes.
- Urine testing must remain an important part of routine health examination for children, especially those who are overweight, because it is often the first clue that a child may have diabetes.

PATIENT 2: A 13-YEAR-OLD MALE WITH MISSED DIAGNOSIS AND FATAL HYPEROSMOLAR STATE

- African-American found to have large glucosuria and ketonuria during a visit to primary physician for routine sports examination
- hypercholesterolemia diagnosed 2 years earlier
- father and older brother with type 2 diabetes
- weight 78 kg, height 157 cm; BMI 32 kg/m^2, nearly 4 SD above the normal for age of 18.5 kg/m^2
- no action taken on urine findings
- vomiting starting the day after the sports examination; after 3 days of persistent emesis, abdominal pain, and malaise, again seen by the physician
  - 3.2-kg weight loss
  - diffusely tender abdomen
  - promethazine suppositories prescribed with advice to increase oral intake of fluids
- 3 days later, found unresponsive, asystolic, and apneic, with fixed dilated pupils
  - resuscitative efforts unsuccessful
  - laboratory serum determinations: glucose 1,083 mg/dl (60 mmol/l), osmolality 377 mEq/l, pH 6.6, potassium 5.9 mEq/l, CO_2 26 mEq/l, 'small' acetone; hematocrit 51%
  - postmortem examination: vitreous glucose concentration 619 mg/dl (34 mmol/l), acute purulent bronchiolitis, cerebral edema, unremarkable microscopic examination of the pancreas

Comments

- With glucosuria, ketonuria, a strong family history of type 2 diabetes, and obesity, this young man had a typical clinical picture for type 2 diabetes.
- Type 2 diabetes can be the cause of acute decompensation, and a high index of suspicion is required to prevent serious morbidity or mortality.
- The finding of glucosuria, especially with ketonuria, is as much an emergency situation in children with type 2 diabetes as in children with type 1 diabetes.
- Although diabetic ketoacidosis at the time of diagnosis is becoming increasingly recognized in type 2 diabetes, when significant hyperglycemia

results in β-cell toxicity with reduced insulin secretion and consequent fat breakdown and ketone formation, there is little appreciation that hyperosmolar coma and cerebral edema can occur in this condition.

■ This patient and Patient 3 are among eight fatalities at onset of type 2 diabetes in children known to the authors; all are the result of failure to act on findings indicating hyperglycemia and severe dehydration or the result of acting inappropriately (Morales A, Rosenbloom AL: Death at the onset of type 2 diabetes [T2DM] in African-American youth. *Pediatr Res.* 51:124A, 2002).

PATIENT 3: A 15-YEAR-OLD MALE WITH HYPEROSMOLAR STATE AND FATAL HYPOKALEMIA

■ African-American given ibuprofen in an emergency room for 3 days of dizziness, lethargy, headaches, and vomiting

■ height normal, weight 107 kg; BMI 31 kg/m², 3.3 SD above normal for age of 19.5 kg/m²

■ seen by personal pediatrician later that day, who prescribed combination of aspirin, butalbital, codeine, and caffeine (Fiorinal)

■ seen again the next day; told to continue taking this medication, eat a soft diet

■ became extremely lethargic and weak 1 day later; taken to a different ER
  ● serum concentrations: glucose 1,800 mg/dl (100 mmol/l), sodium 150 mEq/l, potassium 3.5 mEq/l, CO_2 17 mEq/l, pH 7.25, osmolality 405 mOsm/l
  ● no ketonuria
  ● heart rate 144 beats/minute, BP 137/63 mmHg, respiratory rate 40/minute, Glasgow coma score 13
  ● fluid replacement during the first 2 hours with normal saline
  ● 20 mEq/l potassium chloride then added to IV fluids
  ● 100 mEq sodium bicarbonate given by rapid injection 1 hour later
  ● 10 minutes after the bicarbonate infusion, serum potassium 1.8 mEq/l and multiple rhythm disturbances noted on the electrocardiogram
  ● expired 3 hours later, after a transvenous pacemaker failed to restore normal cardiac rhythm
  ● postmortem findings: mild fatty changes of the liver, no inflammatory changes in the islet cells

Comments

- This patient had headache, lethargy, and vomiting, indicative of increased intracranial pressure.
- Marked hyperglycemia and hyperosmolality, with mild acidosis, were indicative of the hyperglycemic hyperosmolar state.
- The serum potassium concentration of 3.5 mEq/l with pH 7.25 indicates hypokalemia. Each decrease of pH of 0.1 results in an increased serum potassium level of 0.6, as the result of the shift of potassium from the intracellular compartment with acidosis. Thus, the initial corrected potassium value was actually 2.6 mEq/l.
- Vigorous potassium replacement was needed because, as the pH increased with treatment, the potassium level would decrease as potassium ions reentered the cells. Intravenous fluid replacement of 20 mEq/l was not adequate potassium replacement in this instance.
- The hypokalemia was further exacerbated by the rapid injection of sodium bicarbonate, accelerating the correction of acidosis and reentry of potassium into the cells. The sudden shift in pH level and the presence of total body potassium depletion resulted in marked hypokalemia with consequent arrhythmias.
- Children with type 2 diabetes have comparable urinary electrolyte losses as children with type 1 diabetes; the longer duration of hyperglycemia and the resultant osmotic diuresis may result in even more electrolyte depletion in youth with type 2 diabetes.

PATIENT 4: A 13-YEAR-OLD WITH VAGINAL MONILIASIS

- non-Hispanic white seen at a walk-in clinic for a vaginal rash of 10 days duration, diagnosed as candidal vulvovaginitis
- blood glucose tested because of the infection confirmed diabetes
- no polyuria, polydipsia, polyphagia
- referred to hospital
  - A1C 9.5%, blood glucose 440 mg/dl (24.5 mmol/l), β-hydroxybutyrate elevated at 3.1 mg/dl (298 nmol/l)
  - treated with insulin and provided diabetes education
- maternal great grandmother with type 2 diabetes
- inactive at home, playing computer games and listening to music

- height 164 cm, weight 88 kg, BMI 33 kg/m^2, >4 SD above the normal for age of 18.6 kg/m^2
- Tanner stage 5 pubic hair and breast development
- no acanthosis nigricans or hypertension
- A1C reduction to 7.5% during the first 2 months of insulin therapy
- 5 months after diabetes diagnosis, stopped taking insulin because blood glucose levels were always 50–70 mg/dl
  - single self-monitored blood glucose 250 mg/dl ~1 month later
  - injected 2 units regular insulin and blood glucose dropped to 20 mg/dl, with symptoms requiring treatment with glucagon
  - A1C 6.6% 1 month after stopping insulin
  - islet cell antibodies absent, C-peptide level 5.3 pg/l (normal adult range 0.5–2.0)
- insulin restarted
  - further A1C decline to 5.8%
  - advised to decrease portion sizes, drink at least 8 glasses of water/day, exercise daily (did 20 minutes of bike riding/day)
  - decrease in weight from 82.0 to 80.2 kg
- cholesterol 287 mg/dl (7.42 mmol/l) despite excellent metabolic control, treated with statin drug
- metformin 500 mg b.i.d. begun and insulin dose tapered
  - stopped because of nausea and intermittent vomiting
  - insulin dose increased to previous levels
- ~1-1/2 years after diagnosis, diabetes control deteriorated with the development of depression
  - rise in A1C from 6–7% to 9.4%
  - started on enalapril 5 mg b.i.d. for newly developed hypertension
  - decrease in compliance
- admitted to a residential unit for children having difficulty coping with their diabetes
  - lost substantial amount of weight, able to stop all medications for blood glucose control
  - A1C 5.3%, all blood glucose values normal
  - gained 4.5–7.0 kg during 2 months after discharge
- over subsequent year deterioration in compliance
  - checking blood glucose levels 2–5 times per month, only when symptomatic

- not taking any medication for diabetes
- A1C mildly elevated at 6.4%
■ remained off all medication 3 years after diagnosis
  - A1C 7.2%
  - encouraged to establish weight control with diet and exercise with the understanding that if A1C does not decrease, hypoglycemic medication would be needed
  - persistent hypercholesterolemia and hypertension

Comments

■ Vaginitis and dysuria are common clues to type 2 diabetes in adolescents. These findings are often present in the absence of polyuria, polydipsia, or polyphagia, despite substantial hyperglycemia.

■ In these otherwise asymptomatic individuals, treatment with diet and exercise alone may result in sufficient weight loss, causing reversal of the diabetes. However, with longstanding hyperglycemia, as noted in this patient, β-cell toxicity occurs, with reduced insulin secretion, in her case sufficient to result in elevated β-hydroxybutyrate, a reflection of increased lipolysis, which can also contribute to the suppression of insulin secretion. In these instances, initial treatment to decrease glycemia allows endogenous insulin production to resume.

■ Although this patient initially did well, she became noncompliant with insulin injections over time.
  - Because children with type 2 diabetes do not typically or readily develop symptoms of hyperglycemia (polyuria and polydipsia) or ketosis (nausea or vomiting) with discontinuation of their diabetes medications, they are more likely to be noncompliant with medications than are children with type 1 diabetes.
  - Stopping medications may be effective if accompanied by lifestyle changes involving diet and exercise, but in this patient, insulin therapy was stopped without any other changes being made.

■ This patient's hypertension, hypercholesterolemia, and severe documented hyperinsulinism/insulin resistance are likely more important than her relatively mild diabetes.

■ This patient was not a member of what is considered a high-risk ethnic/racial group for childhood type 2 diabetes, emphasizing that membership in such a group is a useful indicator of risk, but that nonmembership should not diminish the high index of suspicion when other risk factors are present.

PATIENT 5: A 13.5-YEAR-OLD FEMALE DEVELOPING KETOACIDOSIS AFTER 6 MONTHS OF NONCOMPLIANCE

- African-American seen in an ER for skin abscess of the face with history of skin abscess of the chest
- glucosuria, trace ketonuria
- no symptoms of diabetes
- obese since 1st grade
- mother obese with acanthosis, obese father dead from an accident, maternal great-grandfather dead from diabetes complications
- normal height for age, weight 131 kg; BMI 50 kg/m², almost 9 SD above normal for age of 19 kg/m²
- acanthosis of neck, axilla, groin; no hirsutism
- Tanner stage 5 development
- no glucosuria on subsequent examination
- random blood glucose 168 mg/dl (9.3 mmol/l), repeat 1-hour postprandial glucose 128 mg/dl (7.1 mmol/l)
- A1C 6.4% (normal for lab 4.1–6.5%).
- intervention
  - education about the risk of type 2 diabetes
  - counseling about diet modification for the whole family
  - encouragement of physical activity
- follow-up
  - several appointments missed in subsequent 6 months
  - in ER with 1 week of vomiting, polyuria, polydipsia, nocturia, headache
    - 15-kg weight loss
    - glucose 621 mg/dl (34.5 mmol/l)
    - pH 7.08, HCO_3 6 mEq/l
    - A1C 13%
  - after treatment of diabetic ketoacidosis, sent home on insulin therapy
- subsequent studies
  - no islet cell or GAD antibodies
  - C-peptide 7 pg/l

- A1C 6.8% on metformin and insulin
- regained all lost weight, BMI remains 50 kg/m²

Comments

- This patient demonstrated typical insidious onset of type 2 diabetes over a 6-month period, with rapid deterioration to typical ketoacidosis.
- Children with new-onset symptomatic type 2 diabetes have similar absolute weight loss as children with type 1 diabetes when groups are compared. Percentage of total body weight lost for those with type 2 diabetes, however, is considerably less than that in children with type 1 diabetes.
- In this family with obese parents, success in attaining weight loss and reducing insulin resistance is not possible unless there is a family commitment to an altered lifestyle.
- Metformin could have been considered for "off-label" use during the 6 months before the development of ketoacidosis to treat acanthosis nigricans and possibly assist in weight reduction.
- Reduction in acanthosis nigricans could have supported compliance and prevention of ketoacidosis.

PATIENT 6: A 15-YEAR-OLD GIRL DIAGNOSED WITH TYPE 1 DIABETES AT 11 YEARS OF AGE

- Caucasian hospitalized at age 11 years for diabetic ketoacidosis
  - polyuria, polydipsia, nocturia for 1–2 months
  - monilial vaginitis
  - A1C 9.9%
  - blood glucose 293 mg/dl (16.3 mmol/l)
  - mother diagnosed with type 1 diabetes at 15 years of age, paternal great-grandfather and maternal grandfather with type 2 diabetes, 2 half-uncles with diabetes of unknown type, a second cousin with type 1 diabetes
  - height 153.6 cm, weight 46.5 kg; BMI 20 kg/m², between 75th and 85th percentile (normal for age 17.5)
  - BP 116/55 mmHg
- A1C 6.8 and 7.9% for 3 years, subsequent deterioration of metabolic control with A1C 9.2%

- urine albumin excretion 157 mg/g creatinine (normal <30 mg/mg creatinine)
- cholesterol 166 mg/dl (4.3 mmol/l), triglycerides 353 mg/dl (4.0 mmol/l), HDL cholesterol 35.5 mg/dl (0.92 mmol/l), LDL cholesterol 60 mg/dl (1.55 mmol/l)
- repeat urine albumin 8 months later normal at 15 mg/g creatinine and again normal 1 year after initial value, at 7 mg/g creatinine
- 4 years after diagnosis (age 15)
  - height 70th percentile but weight 79 kg, BMI 90–95th percentile (27.3 kg/m^2, normal for age 20 kg/m^2) with concern about eating disorder
  - wanted to weigh 60 kg
  - skipped insulin and other medications while taking laxatives and Metabolite to achieve weight loss
  - last menstrual period 1 year previously
- admitted to residential treatment unit for children and adolescents having difficulty coping with their diabetes
  - took 10 units NPH and 5 units regular insulin before breakfast, 15 units regular insulin before supper, 16 units NPH insulin at bedtime
  - frequent hypoglycemia requiring insulin dose reduction to 6 units NPH and 1 unit insulin lispro in the morning, 4 units NPH and 4 units insulin lispro before supper
  - metformin 500 mg b.i.d. begun with hopes of weaning off insulin
  - weaning unsuccessful (hyperglycemia)
  - diagnosis changed to type 2 diabetes, because of persistent normal C-peptide levels (1.2 pg/l, normal 0.5–2.0)
  - discharged on metformin 1000 mg b.i.d. with insulin 7 units NPH and 1 unit insulin lispro in the morning, 3 units NPH and 4 units insulin lispro before supper
- 8 months after discharge from residential unit, weight 78.5 kg, BMI 27.8 kg/m^2 (95th percentile), A1C 10.8%
- stopped insulin 7 weeks before and metformin 4 weeks before next clinic appointment, but gained 0.3 kg since previous visit 4 months earlier
- 4 months later, weight had increased to 83.9 kg and BP to 130/65 mmHg

Comments

- This patient was classified as having type 1 diabetes at diagnosis because of lack of obesity, Caucasian ethnicity, and ketoacidosis.

- Atypical course for type 1 diabetes led to reevaluation of initial diagnosis, emphasizing the fact that, for some patients, correct diagnosis can only be made after observing the clinical course for 1 or more years.
- Reclassification as type 2 diabetes was dictated by:
  - normal fasting C-peptide 4 years after diagnosis
  - ability to discontinue insulin for 7 weeks and oral medication for 3 of those weeks without developing ketoacidosis
- MODY might be considered in the differential diagnosis of this patient with mild overweight at onset and a strong family history of diabetes. Although ketoacidosis does not occur at the onset of MODY, with insulin dependence occurring (if at all) years after diagnosis, it would be of interest to search for MODY mutations or mitochondrial mutations in this patient. Treatment should not depend on absolute classification; rather, it should be determined by the knowledge that fasting C-peptide is normal, obesity is now a complicating factor, and the treatment approach is that for type 2 diabetes.

PATIENT 7: AN 11.5-YEAR-OLD MALE WITH TYPICAL SIGNS AND SYMPTOMS OF DIABETES

- Puerto Rican with polyuria, polydipsia, polyphagia, weight loss
- hospitalized with blood glucose >200 mg/dl (>11 mmol/l)
- height 165 cm, weight 71.2 kg; BMI 26 kg/m^2, 2.8 SD above the normal for age of 17.5 kg/m^2
- diabetes in mother, maternal aunt, maternal grandfather and grandmother, maternal great-grandfather, maternal great uncle, all of whom were obese
- diagnosed with type 2 diabetes because of Hispanic ethnicity, family history, obesity
- 10-kg weight loss with strict diet
- glucose 85–133 mg/dl (4.7–7.4 mmol/l), A1C 4.6% without medication, 10 months after diagnosis
- glucose 92–121 mg/dl (5.1–6.7 mmol/l) preprandial and 121–162 mg/dl (6.7–9.0 mmol/l) postprandial 15 months after diagnosis
  - BP 128/75 mmHg, systolic >90th percentile for age and height
  - 2$^+$ proteinuria
  - A1C 4.5%

Comments

- Despite metabolic decompensation at the time of diagnosis with typical symptoms of diabetes, the patient has thus far (15 months) been able to control his diabetes with a successful weight reduction program.
- Despite good diabetes control, the patient is developing hypertension and proteinuria, which may eventually be a more serious problem for him than his diabetes, again emphasizing that hyperglycemia is only one manifestation of the insulin resistance syndrome.

PATIENT 8: A 7.5-YEAR-OLD BOY WITH HYPEROSMOLAR STATE

- hyperglycemic hyperosmolar state at diagnosis, with blood glucose >1,000 mg/dl (>55 mmol/l)
  - not comatose
  - severely obese African-American
  - hospitalized for 1.5 weeks
  - discharged on 1 unit/kg/day insulin
- strong family history of diabetes, including mother with poorly controlled type 2 diabetes
- A1C 5.9% 1 1/4 years after diagnosis
- did well for 1 3/4 years with reduction in insulin dose to 4 units NPH/day and metformin 500 mg b.i.d.
- weight 118 kg, height 155.5 cm; BMI 49 kg/m^2, 13 SD above the normal for age of 16 kg/m^2
- BP 143/62 mmHg, and later 174/70 mmHg, systolic well above 95th percentile for height (systolic of 119)
- noncompliant with blood glucose monitoring and with taking insulin or oral medications; no parental supervision, with mother allowing him to miss medication
- increasing blood glucose levels after a viral infection 21 months after diagnosis with resultant gradual increase in insulin dose to 40 units NPH, 25 units regular insulin in the morning and 45 units NPH, 20 units regular insulin in the evening
- 2 months later, weight had decreased to 113 kg despite no attempt at dietary restriction or exercise; A1C 14%
- because of persistent noncompliance and failure of supervision, not responsive to outpatient counseling, admitted to residential rehabilitation facility 2 years after diagnosis

- with further 10-kg weight loss, A1C normalized to 5.8%
- able to discontinue all medication and remain euglycemic
- discharge after 5 months in residential unit
- readmission to hospital for hyperosmolality
  - regained 5 kg
  - blood glucose 542 mg/dl (30 mmol/l)
  - A1C 9.36%
  - BP 141/72 mmHg
  - metformin 500 mg b.i.d. and 40 units 70/30 insulin mix reinstituted
- metabolic control remained poor despite increasing 70/30 insulin to 50 units b.i.d., changing metformin regimen to extended formulation (1,000 mg once daily), and adding pioglitazone
- over next 4–5 months, 3 1/12 years after diagnosis, 3 emergency room visits for vomiting and dehydration requiring IV fluids and 1 hospitalization for ketoacidosis, with large urine ketones, blood glucose 799 mg/dl (44.4 mmol/l), Na 127 meq/l, CO_2 11 meq/l, A1C 17.6%, urine protein 2+
- in desperation and concern for the child's welfare, referral made to the state's children and families office for medical neglect, with profound effect of motivating the mother to improve compliance, with subsequent A1C 6.1%

Comments

- Type 2 diabetes can occur in prepubertal children if they are obese and genetically at risk. This child weighed 118 kg (250 lb) at 9 years of age, was of high-risk ethnicity, and had a strong family history of type 2 diabetes.
- Poor metabolic control in the parents of a child with type 2 diabetes is a warning sign that the child, too, is at risk for noncompliance and poor metabolic control.
- Hypertension and proteinuria were noted early in the course of the disease, within the first 3 years after diagnosis. Complications appear to be aggressive in children with type 2 diabetes, and hypertension and hyperlipidemia should be treated early with ACE inhibitors and statins.
- Persistent poor compliance with medical recommendations and failure of counseling, as with type 1 diabetes, may, as a last resort, require referral to a family service agency. It is not uncommon for such a referral to serve as a wake-up call to motivate the family.

- It is imperative to simplify the regimen of children in whom compliance is an issue. In this patient, the use of 70/30 insulin avoided the necessity for mixing insulins, and changing from the twice-daily formulation of metformin to the 24-hour preparation enhanced the likelihood that oral medications would be taken.

PATIENT 9: A 17-YEAR-OLD MALE DIAGNOSED WITH TYPE 1 DIABETES AT 11 YEARS OF AGE

- polyuria and 7-kg weight loss at diagnosis
- tall and obese, with height 166 cm (90th percentile for age), weight 84 kg; BMI 31 kg/m², 4 SD above normal for age of 19 kg/m²
- glucose 530 mg/dl (29.4 mmol/l), pH 7.39, Na 127 mEq/l, CO_2 28 mEq/l
- A1C 13.6%
- insulin 19 μU/mL (136 pmol/l)
- treated with insulin
- mother from the Philippines, father from India
- maternal grandmother, great-grandmother, great-great-grandmother with diabetes of adult onset
- 4 years after initial treatment period, started on metformin with reduction of A1C from 11.1 to 9.8%
- at 17.5 years of age, height 184 cm, weight 143 kg; BMI 40 kg/m², nearly 7 SD above the normal mean of 19.5 kg/m²
  - acanthosis nigricans of the neck
  - C-peptide 2.4 μg/l (normal 0.9-4.0 μg/l)
  - islet cell antibodies >80 JDF units (normal <5 JDF units); GAD antibodies 7.9 units/ml (normal <2.5 units/ml)

Comments

- The initial diagnosis of type 1 diabetes was based on age and severity, with polyuria, weight loss, and high glucose and A1C levels, despite risk factors for type 2 diabetes including ethnicity, obesity, and strong family history of adult diabetes.
- Reassessment 4 years after diagnosis led to consideration of type 2 diabetes and successful introduction of metformin—a step that would have been highly unlikely to be helpful this long after diagnosis of type 1 diabetes.
- Presence of markers of islet autoimmunity 6.5 years after diagnosis causes a diagnostic dilemma, but the evidence for type 1 diabetes is otherwise

very weak, with the elevated plasma insulin concentration at diagnosis and normal C-peptide level 6.5 years after diagnosis entirely inconsistent with type 1 diabetes. Nonetheless, the evidence of autoimmune disease of the islet cells indicates latent type 1 diabetes that has yet to result in sufficient insulin deficiency superimposed on the insulin-resistant type 2 diabetes to require insulin replacement. It is more important to treat the patient than the presumed diabetes classification in the aggressive pursuit of near-normal glycemia.

■ If blood glucose levels do not reach target goals on maximal dose of metformin and compliance is ensured, a second agent will need to be added, and if this is ineffective in achieving blood glucose goals, insulin may be needed.

About the American Diabetes Association

The American Diabetes Association is the nation's leading voluntary health organization supporting diabetes research, information, and advocacy. Its mission is to prevent and cure diabetes and to improve the lives of all people affected by diabetes. The American Diabetes Association is the leading publisher of comprehensive diabetes information. Its huge library of practical and authoritative books for people with diabetes covers every aspect of self-care—cooking and nutrition, fitness, weight control, medications, complications, emotional issues, and general self-care.

To order American Diabetes Association books: Call 1-800-232-6733. Or log on to http://store.diabetes.org

To join the American Diabetes Association: Call 1-800-806-7801. www.diabetes.org/membership

For more information about diabetes or ADA programs and services: Call 1-800-342-2383. E-mail: AskADA@diabetes.org or log on to www.diabetes.org

To locate an ADA/NCQA Recognized Provider of quality diabetes care in your area: www.ncqa.org/dprp/

To find an ADA Recognized Education Program in your area: Call 1-888-232-0822. www.diabetes.org/recognition/education.asp

To join the fight to increase funding for diabetes research, end discrimination, and improve insurance coverage: Call 1-800-342-2383. www.diabetes.org/advocacy

To find out how you can get involved with the programs in your community: Call 1-800-342-2383. See below for program Web addresses.

- *American Diabetes Month:* Educational activities aimed at those diagnosed with diabetes—month of November. www.diabetes.org/ADM
- *American Diabetes Alert:* Annual public awareness campaign to find the undiagnosed—held the fourth Tuesday in March. www.diabetes.org/alert
- *The Diabetes Assistance & Resources Program (DAR):* Diabetes awareness program targeted to the Latino community. www.diabetes.org/DAR
- *African American Program:* Diabetes awareness program targeted to the African American community. www.diabetes.org/africanamerican
- *Awakening the Spirit: Pathways to Diabetes Prevention & Control:* Diabetes awareness program targeted to the Native American community. www.diabetes.org/awakening

To find out about an important research project regarding type 2 diabetes: www.diabetes.org/ada/research.asp

To obtain information on making a planned gift or charitable bequest: Call 1-888-700-7029. www.diabetes.org/ada/plan.asp

To make a donation or memorial contribution: Call 1-800-342-2383. www.diabetes.org/ada/cont.asp